The Signs and Symptoms of Menopause

A Vital Book for Women Exploring Perimenopause, Postmenopause, HRT Therapy, Hot Flashes, Night Sweats, Weight Gain, and Other Menopause Symptoms

I0092494

Rachel Wright

Thank You!

Thank you for your purchase.

I am dedicated to making the most enriching and informational content. I hope it meets your expectations and you gain a lot from it.

INTRODUCTION

It's not just about irregular periods and hot flashes. Menopause is a time of new beginnings. It's a time for you to take charge of your life and do what you want, when you want, and how you want. Women experience a range of health changes in the years before and after menopause. When you understand and prepare for this transition, you'll move through it more easily.

There's no reason to let menopause get in the way of your life or even your dreams.

Did you know that menopause is a natural part of aging?

Yep! And it's not just "hormonal changes"— it's a whole new chapter in your life.

So why do so many women feel like they're going crazy when they hit their 40s and beyond?

Menopause is a mystery to many women, and we are rarely prepared for it. I created this book because of the stigma associated with women's health and how we talk about it. I want to make sure that every woman has access to genuine, compassionate care for herself and her family. I have met many women who do not fully understand the changes that this time of hormone fluctuation can bring or how long such symptoms may last. Yes, they all know about flushes and irregular periods. Still, many women worry about other symptoms like mood changes, itching, tiredness, bladder symptoms, and poor memory, unaware that these can also be linked to menopausal changes. They want to understand menopause, its effects on the body, and the different options for symptom relief, both medical and non-medical.

Menopause is a time of incredible change and freedom. It's also a time when women often worry about what's happening to them and how they will manage their lives. It can be difficult to know what to expect.

You may have heard that menopause means a woman's body stops making eggs, and her periods stop. That's true, but it's not the whole story. Menopause is a natural process that happens over several years. During this time, your hormones change, affecting your body in many ways. For instance, it causes the cessation of menstruation and the end of fertility. Menopause occurs when the ovaries stop producing estrogen, a hormone needed for egg maturation and ovulation. Due to a decrease in hormone production, changes begin happening in the body, resulting in symptoms like hot flashes, irregular periods, mood swings, and night sweats.

Menopause does not occur overnight; it takes several

years for your hormones to decline to low enough levels until you are no longer fertile. The average age of menopause is 51, but it can occur as early as the mid-40s or as late as the 60s.

The good news is you can do many things to stay healthy during menopause!

Menopause is a natural part of life, not a disease. It can be an exciting time, as well as a challenging one. The body goes through this transition every month, and many changes occur during this time in your life (both physically and emotionally). These changes can sometimes make you feel less like yourself and more like an alien! The good news is that there are many ways to deal with these symptoms and make the transition easier for your body and mind.

Menopause can be challenging for many women, but it does not have to be difficult or stressful. Getting through menopause can be one of the hardest times in your life. It's confusing, it's emotional, and it's not fun. However, if you know what to expect and how to handle it, you can make this transition easier on yourself—and be ready to take on whatever comes next!

Women today are busy. We have family and friends, work, social commitments, and more. When we reach menopause, it can feel like we're entering a new stage of our lives that requires special care and attention, and we wonder how we'll find the time for all that. But don't worry! This book makes it easy to find the supports you need to get through this time of change with ease and grace. Here you'll find approaches that work for you with complete explanations of what's happening and why.

Women often feel alone during their menopause years, and many search the internet to find online articles for the information they need to make informed choices. Knowing what's true online and what's not can be difficult. This book aims to fill the gap, providing practical information about menopause, explaining what is normal, and giving you tools to cope with it all. It will help you understand that there is more to this transition than simply discontinuing periods and aims to equip you with everything you need to get through this critical time. This book provides a helpful guide for women approaching or who have already entered menopause. It will help you understand what is happening with your body and offers practical strategies for dealing with day-to-day challenges such as hot flashes, night sweats, mood swings, memory loss, vaginal dryness, or pain during sex. This book also helps women navigate the process of transitioning from being a mother/carer to being an individual again as they start living anew after years of being busy raising children (or caring for someone else).

This book will explore the following:

- A stage-by-stage summary of health changes most women experience
- What's happening in your body as it changes during menopause
- Symptoms that can occur around menopause, including hot flashes, vaginal dryness, and mood swings
- An overview of medical conditions that can occur during menopause and after, with self-tests to help you assess your risks

- Managing menopause at work
- Breaking the bias and stigma about menopause
- Tips on lifestyle choices and complementary therapies to care for your body, mind, and relationships.

Menopause is a transition. Your midlife years—before, during, and after menopause can be a positive time, even if you face some health challenges. It's normal to feel scared, confused, and anxious about what's happening in your body. While you're going through menopause, it's important to remember that you are still YOU! You don't have to change yourself or give up your interests just because you're going through this transition.

The best way to deal with the symptoms of menopause is to stay informed about what's happening with your body. Menopause can cause unpleasant side effects, but they are temporary and should improve over time as your hormones adjust. Menopause doesn't need to be a scary time—it's an exciting time for many women because it means they're entering a new stage of life!

Whether your menopause transition is smooth or

challenging, this book is for you, as taking excellent care of your health through these years is more essential than ever. You'll feel better now and be able to age more gracefully.

Whether you're on the rollercoaster of menopause or just beginning to think about it, this book is for you!

Whether you see menopause as a natural event that does not need medical intervention or whether you are seeking all the medical help available for symptom relief, this book is for you!

Let's begin!

CHAPTER 1: THE MENOPAUSE TRANSITION

Menopause is a natural part of life, but it can be an uncomfortable and sometimes scary experience. The good news is that you're not alone! Menopause will happen to all women, so it's essential to understand and learn how to manage the transition.

What is Menopause?

The term "menopause" is commonly used to mean the entire transition women go through in the years before, during, and after their last menstrual period. Menopause is a time in a woman's life when her

15

ovaries stop producing eggs, and she stops having a monthly period.

It's a normal part of aging but also a time when you may experience changes in your body and emotions. These changes can be hard to deal with, but there are things you can do to help manage them. You may have heard that menopause is caused by low estrogen levels, which is true. However, it's also true that you can have high estrogen levels during menopause if your ovaries are still releasing eggs.

During the menopause transition, you may have periods that are heavier than usual or shorter, and some women don't have periods at all anymore, or they skip a month or two. Menopause proper is diagnosed after a woman goes a full 12 months with no menstrual periods.

You may be done with periods, but menopause doesn't mean that you're done with sex! You can still enjoy intimacy with your partner even if you do not have periods anymore. In fact, it is a time of tremendous freedom because you no longer have to worry about using contraception or getting pregnant. Do remember, though, that you still need to practice safe sex to prevent infections. Things may become a little dry down below, but this is easily solved.

Why does Menopause occur?

Menopause is caused by naturally declining reproductive hormones and the ovaries' decline in egg cells. Menopause occurs naturally when a woman's ovaries run out of functioning eggs. As you approach your late 30s and beyond, your ovaries start making less estrogen and progesterone — the hormones that regulate menstruation — and your fertility declines. As a result, your body will stop menstruating, and you'll experience other symptoms that come with menopause, such as hot flashes and night sweats. Menopause can also occur if certain diseases or cancer treatments damage a woman's ovaries or if they are surgically removed.

Stages of Menopause

There are three stages of menopause: perimenopause, menopause, and postmenopause. Those names can be

17

translated into simpler terms: when changes begin, when your menstrual cycle stops, and your new normal afterward. Here's a closer look at what happens during each one.

Perimenopause

The beginning of menopause. Perimenopause is when your body starts transitioning towards menopause, and symptoms begin. It is when your body starts to go through changes in hormone levels that will lead up to your last period. This stage typically begins about 4-8 years before true menopause. During this time, your hormones fluctuate, and you might experience symptoms like hot flashes or night sweats. You may also have vaginal dryness, mood swings, and other symptoms depending on how far along you are in perimenopause. Menstrual periods become shorter and lighter or more prolonged and heavier. The interval between periods becomes unpredictable. These changes happen because your body's estrogen and progesterone levels gradually decline. As your ovaries produce lower amounts of these hormones, your body adapts. It's the reverse of what happened to your hormones as a teenager. Perimenopause typically

18

occurs in your 40's with an average age of 47.

Menopause

The end of your menstrual cycle. Menopause is the final menstrual period and is confirmed when a woman has not had her period for 12 consecutive months. Reaching menopause means that you're no longer able to become pregnant. All women, except those whose ovaries were removed, will go through menopause. During this period, the ovaries no longer release eggs and no longer secrete estrogen and progesterone. Menopause typically occurs between the ages of 40-55, with an average age of 51.

Postmenopause

Life after menopause. Postmenopause refers to the stage after menopause when it's been 12 months or more since your last period. Postmenopause signals the end of your reproductive years, and you'll be in this stage for the rest of your life. During this phase, symptoms begin to ease or disappear. Postmenopause typically starts in your early to mid-50s.

Premature and Early Menopause

Premature menopause is when a woman's final menstrual period occurs before she is 40 years of age.

Early menopause is when a woman's final menstrual period occurs between the ages of 40 and 45.

This happens when the body unexpectedly stops producing female hormones (estrogen and progesterone).

It occurs in about 1% of women and is often caused by one of the following:

- Hysterectomy
- Thyroid problems
- Surgical menopause
- Endometrial cancer
- Ovarian torsion (tearing of the ovaries)
- Chemotherapy
- Radiation treatment
- Autoimmune disorders

There is no cure for early menopause, but some treatments can help alleviate some of its symptoms. These include hormone therapy using estrogen pills or patches, lifestyle changes like losing weight if you are overweight, quitting smoking if you smoke, moderate exercise such as walking 30 minutes daily, and avoiding caffeine, including coffee.

Can You Get Pregnant during Perimenopause?

Yes, you can get pregnant during perimenopause, but it's less likely and a little more complicated. You may have irregular periods or no periods during this time, but your body is still producing eggs. Your body will also still ovulate (release an egg). However, there are some risks associated with pregnancy during perimenopause. Pregnancy complications like gestational diabetes and high blood pressure are more likely to occur during this time than during any other part of your reproductive life span.

The hormones released by your body during pregnancy—including estrogen, progesterone, and relaxin—are different from those released during other points in your life cycle as well because they change as you age into menopause. These changes can affect how much blood flow is available for your baby's development inside the womb (uterus).

Although pregnancy is less likely around menopause, it is still important to use contraception until menopause has been confirmed if you wish to avoid an unplanned pregnancy.

During perimenopause, a woman's periods may become irregular and unpredictable. However, her ovaries are still likely to be producing some eggs, so though natural fertility does decline, pregnancy can happen.

Additionally, research has shown that women who conceive during perimenopause tend to have babies with lower birth weights than those who conceive at other times. This could be due to decreased blood flow or a lack of hormones. There is also an increased likelihood (1 in 100) of conceiving a Down's syndrome baby after the age of 40.

What Are the First Signs of Menopause?

The first signs of menopause are often subtle. You may notice a change in your cycle, such as an increase or decrease in the time between periods. You may also experience changes in the flow or consistency of your period, including heavier or lighter flow, longer or shorter bleeding times, and spotting before or after your period.

You may also experience hot flashes during the first year after your last menstrual period. Some women experience them only occasionally, while others experience them more frequently. Hot flashes can last a few seconds to several minutes at a time.

What Happens When You Are in Menopause?

Menopause is the time in a woman's life when her menstrual cycle stops. This can be stressful for many women because it marks the end of fertility and can make sex much less enjoyable. When you're in menopause, your body no longer produces the hormones it needs to keep your reproductive system

23

running smoothly.

When you're in menopause, you will experience various changes in your body. These changes can include hot flashes and night sweats, vaginal dryness and soreness, skin changes such as dryness or itching, and mood swings. The good news is that these symptoms are temporary—so don't worry!

Skin changes like wrinkles, loss of elasticity in the face (like sagging jowls!), thinning hair on the scalp (called alopecia), and thinning nails may also occur during this time of life cycle change.

How Long Does Menopause Last?

Menopause refers to a specific point in time when your periods stop. You're only in the menopause stage for one year because when you've gone 12 consecutive months without a period, you enter postmenopause. However, the symptoms of menopause can begin several years before a woman's final period and continue for a few years afterward.

The menopausal transition most often begins between

ages 45 and 55. It usually lasts about seven years but can be as long as 14. The duration can depend on lifestyle factors such as smoking, the age it starts, and ethnicity. The menopausal transition affects each woman uniquely and in various ways. Perimenopausal symptoms last four years on average. The symptoms associated with this phase will gradually ease during menopause and postmenopause.

Symptoms of Menopause

The symptoms of menopause are different for everyone, and they can vary from year to year in the same woman. Some women experience very few or even no symptoms at all. However, for others, it can be a difficult transition as their bodies adjust to the changes that come with this stage of life.

The most common symptoms include the following:

Irregular menstruation

As estrogen levels drop, the menstrual cycle changes. You may miss periods or experience more time between periods. Your bleeding may become lighter or heavier. If you're worried or uncertain about your bleeding, I recommend keeping notes on your cycles for a few months. If you're still concerned after that, visit your gynecologist.

Hot flashes

Hot flashes are one of the most common menopausal symptoms. Hot flashes occur when your body overheats because of a drop in estrogen levels. They feel like intense flushing accompanied by sweating and often cause you to feel uncomfortably warm or even break out in a sweat while sleeping at night. Hot flashes can happen any time during the day or night, but they typically occur when your body is resting—like when you're relaxing on the couch or sitting at your desk at work. Hot flashes that happen while you're sleeping are called *night sweats*. Sometimes night sweats can be strong enough to wake you up.

Sleep problems

Sleep problems are another common symptom experienced by many women as they go through menopause. Some women find it hard to fall asleep or stay asleep throughout the night, while others

26

experience vivid dreams or nightmares and wake up feeling unrested no matter how long they sleep each night.

Weight gain

Metabolism tends to slow during menopause, which may cause sudden weight changes.

Bloating

Many women experience bloating during menopause for several reasons. They may experience water retention, gassiness, or slower digestion due to stress.

Joint pain

Estrogen helps decrease inflammation and keep the joints lubricated. As a result, some females experience joint pain due to reduced estrogen levels.

Thinning skin and hair

Extreme fluctuations in hormone levels might cause the skin to become thinner. Some women may experience hair loss.

Changes in sex drive

Menopause also affects libido or desire for sex. It is common to lose interest in and pleasure from sex during menopause. This can directly result from lower levels of testosterone and estrogen, making physical arousal more difficult.

Vaginal symptoms

Vaginal dryness is another common symptom of menopause that affects many women at some point during this transition. This happens because estrogen levels drop as your body transitions into menopause, which can cause your vaginal tissue to become thinner and drier than normal. To manage vaginal dryness, use lubricant during intercourse or masturbation (if not using condoms). Other vaginal symptoms can include:

- Itching and irritation
- Vaginal discharge
- Discomfort or pain during sex with penetration

Mood swings or emotional changes

Feelings of sadness or irritability are common in women going through menopause, especially during

28

the first year after their last period. These emotional changes can be caused by hormonal changes in the brain as well as changes in estrogen levels throughout the body.

Difficulty concentrating

A decline in estrogen can sometimes cause mental fogginess or difficulty concentrating. Menopause can also affect memory.

These symptoms can be uncomfortable, but most women find that they improve over time. Talk to your doctor if your symptoms are affecting your life or if you are concerned about them. They will be able to advise you on treatments that could help relieve your symptoms or recommend alternative treatments such as hormone replacement therapy (HRT). Though there's still stigma and embarrassment around menopause, it's essential to know that you're not alone and there's support out there.

Try to be open about your symptoms with your partner, family, and friends – it can help them understand what you're going through and reduce any embarrassment about symptoms such as sweating.

Sharing experiences with other women going through the same thing could be reassuring. There are many websites, articles, and videos online where women have shared their stories of menopause.

Complications of Menopause

After menopause, women live with long-term hormone deficiency for the rest of their lives. When it comes to a lack of estrogen, the two most significant impacts on your health in the future are the risk of your bones weakening and the risk of disease in your heart and blood vessels. Your risk of certain medical conditions increases. Examples include:

Osteoporosis

There are several possible complications related to menopause. One of them is osteoporosis. It is a condition that causes bones to become fragile and weak.

Heart Disease

Other complications are heart disease and high blood pressure. Many women are affected by these health issues during menopause because they have higher estrogen levels than other women of their age group, which can put them at risk for developing these conditions.

Type 2 Diabetes

Another complication is type 2 diabetes because estrogen helps regulate blood sugar levels in the body. As women enter menopause, they may notice that their blood sugar levels are not as stable as they were when they were younger, which can lead to diabetes later on down the road if left untreated.

Urinary Problems

Urinary incontinence (the occasional and involuntary release of urine) is common in aging women, particularly after menopause. The decline in estrogen causes the vaginal tissues and lining of the urethra to thin out and lose elasticity. As a result, you may experience uncontrollable urine leakage. This often occurs during sudden movements, such as laughing or coughing.

Sexual function

Vaginal dryness from decreased moisture production and loss of elasticity can cause discomfort and slight bleeding during sexual intercourse. Also, decreased sensation may reduce your desire for sexual activity

Depression

The hormone changes in menopause can trigger depression, especially if you have a personal or family history of it. Even if you have not had problems with depression in the past, the stresses and hormone shifts at this time of life can overwhelm your ability to cope. Sometimes the combination of situations and hormones will send you into depression despite your best efforts to manage your mood. If you feel this way, speak with your healthcare provider.

How is Menopause Diagnosed?

Signs and symptoms of menopause are usually enough to tell most women that they've started the menopausal transition. If you have concerns about irregular periods or hot flashes, talk with your doctor. In some cases, further evaluation may be recommended.

There are several ways your healthcare provider can diagnose menopause. The first is discussing your menstrual cycle over the last year. Menopause is diagnosed based on a woman's symptoms and physical changes. Tests typically aren't needed to diagnose menopause; however, a doctor may also conduct blood tests to rule out other health conditions that could cause similar symptoms. The doctor will also ask about your medical history, including previous surgeries or hormone treatments.

4 Essential Health Tests for Menopausal Women

Here are four important health tests for menopausal women:

Vitamin D test

It is essential to take care of yourself more than ever

33

during menopause by having regular health checks. A critical test to have during menopause is a vitamin D level check, which can help determine whether you are suffering from a deficiency. Deficiency in vitamin D may cause several issues, including weight gain, depression, and lack of energy. You can easily treat this deficiency by having your doctor prescribe vitamin D3 supplements for you or ensure that you get out into the midday sun for 10 to 30 minutes each week without sunscreen (don't burn, however!) and with some skin exposed.

Vitamin D can help reduce the symptoms of menopause, including hot flashes and night sweats. It also helps to maintain bone health during this time in a woman's life. If you are experiencing any symptoms of menopause, talk to your doctor about getting your vitamin D levels checked. It's a simple blood test.

Bone Density Test

This test measures how strong your bones are by looking at their density—a higher density means more bone mass and less chance of osteoporosis later on in life! If your doctor recommends it, ask for this test before starting any hormone replacement therapy (HRT) treatment so you can monitor the effects on your bones before making any big decisions about HRT treatments.

Cholesterol and Blood pressure

If you're a woman in menopause, you should be getting your cholesterol and blood pressure checked regularly. If you're over 40, it's recommended that you have these tests done at least once every two years. If you're over 50, it's recommended that you have them done every year. If your heart disease and stroke risk factors are elevated, you may need to get these tests more frequently.

If your doctor finds that your cholesterol levels are high or your blood pressure is too high, they may recommend lifestyle changes like diet and exercise to lower the numbers. If those don't work and the numbers remain high, they may recommend medication to help bring them down.

Thyroid Scan

Another essential test for menopause is the thyroid

35

scan. This test helps doctors determine whether your body is producing enough of the hormone thyroxine (T4), which is made by your thyroid gland, or if it's making too much or too little. It also shows whether you have any nodules on your thyroid gland and if you have an overactive or underactive thyroid gland.

Thyroid scans are often done as part of a routine check-up because they can help to diagnose other problems that could be causing your symptoms, such as adrenal insufficiency or hypothyroidism.

Symptom Relief and Treatment

Menopause requires no medical treatment because it is a natural process. Instead, interventions focus on relieving your signs and symptoms and preventing or managing chronic conditions that may occur with this transition. These may include:

Hormone Therapy

Hormone replacement therapy, or HRT, is the most common intervention for menopause. It involves taking estrogen and progesterone together or separately to replace your body's low or missing hormones. It is available as tablets, skin patches, gels, or sprays. HRT is mostly considered a safe and effective treatment for most women going through menopause and perimenopause.

HRT therapy can help you manage symptoms like hot flashes, night sweats, and vaginal dryness or irritation. It's important to talk to your doctor about all of the risks and benefits before starting this therapy.

Antidepressants

Although prescription antidepressants were developed to treat depression and anxiety, we've learned that specific antidepressants reduce some menopause symptoms. They can be an effective alternative to HRT in very low doses with few or no adverse side effects. These medications are called SSRIs/SSNRIs (selective serotonin reuptake inhibitors). Talk with your doctor about which antidepressants may be helpful to ease menopause symptoms.

Natural remedies

Many natural remedies can help ease menopausal

37

symptoms—including soy-based foods, black cohosh, and other herbs, vitamin E supplements, omega-3 fatty acids found in fatty fish like salmon and mackerel, and flaxseed oil capsules or ground flaxseeds added to your daily diet.

One of the best natural remedies is to drink green tea. Green tea is high in antioxidants and helps to boost your metabolism. It also has anti-inflammatory properties, which help reduce symptoms like hot flashes and night sweats. Another great natural remedy is eating foods rich in phytoestrogens, such as soybeans, flaxseeds, and peanut butter (1 tbsp per day). Phytoestrogens bind to estrogen receptors in the body, helping to keep them occupied so that the body does not produce as much estrogen on its own. However, if you're using natural remedies rather than prescription medications to treat your menopausal symptoms, talk to your doctor before taking them regularly because they may interact poorly with other medications or cause an allergic reaction. "Natural" doesn't always mean the treatment is safe or effective.

You can also try acupuncture or yoga to relieve hot

flashes and other symptoms associated with menopause.

Lifestyle changes

Many studies show that making healthier choices helps women move through menopause with more ease, improved health, and less discomfort. The benefits of healthier choices, mind-body methods, self-care, and complementary therapies can continue long beyond your menopause transition. You can use them whether or not you also decide to try hormone therapy.

Lifestyle changes to consider include:

- Healthy diet
- Stop smoking
- Lower alcohol consumption
- 30 minutes of daily exercise
- Healthy weight management
- Annual mammogram
- Stress management
- Meditation
- Talk with friends going through menopause, or join a support group

- Journaling
- Massage therapy

Cognitive Behavioral Therapy (CBT)

CBT is a talking therapy recommended for low mood associated with menopause. It focuses on changing how you think and behave, with sessions in groups or one-on-one with a therapist. You can be referred via your GP, but many women find it is quicker to organize privately.

Menopause Myths

- **Menopause begins at 50** – No, menopause is the last menstrual period. As mentioned earlier, the average age for menopause is 51, but menopause can happen before or after this age. Women may experience perimenopausal symptoms before they have their last period. These symptoms may start a few months, or up to 13 years in some cases, before menopause

- **You will probably gain weight during menopause** – The lowering levels of estrogen can lead to reduced muscle mass, meaning that the body no longer needs as many daily calories as previously. As stated earlier, weight gain can be prevented by following a healthy diet and regular exercise. Focusing on building or maintaining muscle mass through weight training or load-bearing exercise will also help.

- **There's no difference between surgical and natural menopause** – Surgical and natural menopauses are, in fact, very different. When a woman undergoes a total hysterectomy, she will experience an immediate and significant change in hormonal balance rather than the usual more gradual change in natural menopause.

- **The first sign of menopause is a hot flash** – Symptoms in the peri-menopause are varied, and a hot flash may not be the first sign that your body is entering this stage of your life. Tiredness, anxiety, irritability, mood swings, depression, weight gain, hair loss, cravings, poor concentration, forgetfulness, irregular periods, heavy or light periods, and lowered sex drive can all be symptoms of peri-menopause. With so many different possibilities, many women don't recognize their symptoms as being due to the start of menopause.

- **After menopause, you no longer produce hormones** – This is incorrect. During menopause, estrogen and progesterone levels do decrease, but they continue to be produced, just in smaller amounts post-menopause

- **Menopause only causes physical symptoms** – As seen previously, menopause doesn't only cause physical symptoms. Many women also experience psychological symptoms such as anxiety, depression, forgetfulness, and poor memory. Some of these symptoms can be exacerbated by physical symptoms such as night sweats and hot flashes.

- **The only way to get through menopause is HRT** – For many women, self-help approaches are enough to allow them to manage the symptoms of menopause confidently. Being aware of your options is essential in ensuring your mental and physical well-being during and after menopause. Talk to your doctor about your symptoms and choices.

CHAPTER 2: THE MIND

Menopause doesn't just affect your body—it also affects your brain. It is reported that menopausal women show decreased cognitive performance, especially regarding memory, executive function, and processing speed.

How Menopause Affects Brain Function

As we age, many of us notice that our minds are not as sharp as they used to be. This happens for many reasons—we're less likely to exercise regularly, we're more likely to be sleep-deprived, and we're more likely to have high blood pressure or other conditions that

43

can negatively affect the brain. One major factor in the mental decline in women is menopause.

The level of estrogen produced by the ovaries affects brain health in several ways:

- It helps regulate moods and emotions (this is why many women experience mood swings during menopause)
- It helps maintain cognitive function and memory (this includes the ability to learn new things)
- It helps prevent memory loss by keeping arteries clear and healthy

What happens with our brains?

Our brains change during this transition as estrogen levels start to drop and progesterone levels increase. These changes have a significant impact on how well our brains work.

As estrogen levels decrease, the brain undergoes structural changes in its outer layer (the cortex), making it harder for us to remember things or think

44

clearly. In addition, progesterone increases during menopause; this can cause symptoms like hot flashes and night sweats that keep us awake at night—making it even more difficult for us to focus on tasks that require concentration!

So what can we do about all this? Many women report feeling more anxious or depressed during menopause—these mood issues can also make it harder for us to concentrate on tasks.

The brain is the most complex organ in the human body. It's also one of the most malleable. As we age, our brains can change and adapt in several ways. We can learn new things, create new skills and behaviors, and even grow new neurons! However, as you get older, some changes happen to your brain that might not be so positive. One of these changes is due to menopause.

During menopause, levels of estrogen and progesterone decrease significantly—but this doesn't mean that your brain isn't still changing!

One way in which your brain can rewire itself is by forming new connections between neurons called dendrites. These connections allow your brain to process information more efficiently and make sense of what's happening around you. If you've been experiencing menopause symptoms, it's essential to know that your brain can rewire itself in response to changes in hormone levels. One way the brain does this is by activating new pathways to compensate for losing other pathways. This means that your brain can adapt so that you can still perform tasks, even if the hormone changes have made those tasks more difficult.

However, if you're experiencing severe problems with memory or concentration, it might be helpful to talk to your doctor about taking medication.

Psychological Impact of Menopause

Psychological and emotional symptoms such as depression, anxiety, poor concentration, mood swings, irritability, forgetfulness, and sadness are all common during the menopausal period.

The psychological effect of physical symptoms is important too. For many women, a hot flush may be a relatively minor inconvenience that will pass in time. Still, for others, the distress, shame, and negative thoughts that engender around being out of control, embarrassed, and a feeling of aging may mean that they resent the symptoms and suffer psychological distress. Such symptoms may be especially difficult for women who work in close contact with other people all day.

The critical thing to realize when considering the psychological and emotional symptoms of menopause is that they are real. There can be a tendency to dismiss mental health problems, and when the reasons for the issues can be unclear and complex, treatment options may not be easy and will vary according to the individual.

Brain Fog

The average woman experiences a dip in her mental health during menopause. You might struggle to focus on simple tasks or remember things that happened just minutes ago. It's called "brain fog," It can make you feel like you've got cotton balls in your head. While this isn't a permanent condition, it can last for weeks—and sometimes even months—at a time. So what do you do? Well, the first step is figuring out why it's happening.

Menopause can cause memory or concentration problems, making it harder to think clearly and remember things. It's normal, but it can make you feel like your brain has slowed down.

Some people blame hormone changes for their brain fog, but that doesn't tell the whole story. While fluctuating estrogen levels can cause some symptoms of brain fog, they're not always to blame—and other factors are at play too.

For example, stress! When stressed, your brain tends to take a hit—especially regarding memory and concentration skills. That's because stress affects your brain's ability to perform new tasks and retain information for later use.

Anxiety

The transition to menopause can be an incredibly stressful time for many women. The stress that comes with these changes can also provoke anxiety in women. In fact, according to the American Psychological Association (APA), anxiety is one of the most common symptoms of menopause, and many things can cause it:

- Changes in hormones
- Lack of sleep or poor sleep quality
- Stressful life events

Anxiety, or the feeling of being worried and nervous, is a common symptom during menopause. Because anxiety is difficult to avoid, it's essential to know how to manage it.

You may find that your mood swings between periods of intense worry and relaxation. This can make you feel like you're going crazy! Luckily, there are ways to deal with anxiety symptoms during menopause.

Some easy ways to deal with anxiety include:

- Practice deep breathing exercises
- Try yoga or meditation
- Take time for yourself every day (for example, go for a walk or read a book)

Depression

The symptoms of depression and menopause overlap, making it difficult to know whether you're experiencing one, the other, or both. Both conditions can cause changes in your mood, energy level, sleep patterns, appetite, and concentration.

Depression is a condition that can affect anyone, regardless of gender or age. Depression is a mental health condition that causes feelings of sadness and hopelessness. These feelings can interfere with your daily life, work, or relationships. Both depression and menopause are widespread conditions that can happen at the same time in some people. About half of women with depression also experience menopause-related symptoms at some point.

In some cases, women going through menopause are more likely to experience depression than those who aren't. However, it's important to realize that just because something is linked doesn't mean one causes the other. For example, stress can make you more likely to get sick, but stress doesn't cause illness—it just increases the chances of an illness developing.

What does this mean for menopausal women? It means that if you're already dealing with depression before you go through menopause, you should be aware that your symptoms may get worse when experiencing hormonal changes in your body. You should seek help from your doctor or therapist to address whatever issues result from these changes.

Anger

It's normal to feel frustrated, upset, and angry during a time of change, such as menopause. It is important to remember that you can control your anger and choose how to express it.

During menopause, it can be hard to manage your anger. At this time, you may feel frustrated and angry at others for no apparent reason. This is because you are dealing with many physical and emotional changes that can be difficult to navigate. The good news is that there are some things you can do to help yourself cope with these feelings of frustration and anger.

You should remember that it is perfectly normal to feel angry during menopause. Your body is going through many changes, which can be frustrating when things don't go exactly how you want them to. If you find yourself feeling frustrated or angry, try taking some time for yourself to relax and calm down before interacting with others again. It will help you focus on what needs to be done instead of worrying about other things like anger or frustration over something small like traffic jams or lines at the store!

It's important to know that your anger is valid and normal—but it's also important not to let it take over your life or destroy meaningful relationships. Anger can become a problem when it turns into rage and violence or when you turn your anger inward and become depressed. Anger can make us feel like we're losing control of our lives and our emotions. We know this isn't easy—but we also know it's possible to get help for your anger issues if you want it.

Sleeplessness

Sleeplessness is a common problem for women going through menopause. Many women report that they experience more sleepless nights as they approach menopause. It's not just about getting enough sleep— it's also about the quality of sleep. Menopausal women tend to have more trouble falling asleep and staying asleep. They often wake up feeling tired because their body hasn't had enough time to get into the deeper stages of sleep, which are the most restorative parts of the night. Some things that can help with this include changing your routine (e.g., avoiding caffeine and alcohol before bed), trying yoga or meditation, and making sure your bedroom is dark and quiet enough to promote restful sleep.

For some women, this sleeplessness is caused by hot flashes or night sweats. For others, it's the result of hormonal fluctuations that make it difficult to fall asleep at night and wake up in the morning. Whatever the cause, it's important to treat this disorder promptly before you start developing other health problems.

Here are some tips for managing sleep during menopause:

1. Try to get at least eight hours of sleep every night and avoid naps during the day—this will help regulate your circadian rhythm and improve your overall health. Other women find it helpful to sleep less at night but take time for a short "power nap'" in the afternoon. Find what works best for you.

2. Make sure you're eating right—it's essential to eat plenty of protein and complex carbs before bedtime so that these foods don't interfere with your sleep cycle (you can try eating them earlier in the day instead). Also, ensure you're drinking lots of water throughout the day so that dehydration won't keep you from getting restful sleep later on!

3. Exercise regularly helps reduce stress hormones that might keep you awake at night.

4. Sleep in a cool room with good air circulation.

5. Take a warm bath or shower before bedtime to induce relaxation.

6. Drink warm milk or have a small bowl of yogurt for dessert in the evening. Dairy products contain tryptophan, an amino acid that has a role in serotonin and melatonin production.

7. Chamomile tea before bedtime may also help you to sleep better because it contains apigenin, an antioxidant that binds to specific brain receptors and promotes sleepiness.

8. Almonds are a source of melatonin, a hormone that tells your body it's time to sleep. A handful of these after supper may encourage better sleep.

Stress

Stress is a complex topic—it can be physical, psychological, or even social. However, it's also something we all deal with in one way or another. You've probably heard that stress can cause headaches or ulcers, but did you know it can also lead to menopause?

Stress can cause early menopause. It can also affect your menstrual cycle and make you more likely to have irregular periods. There are several ways that stress contributes to early menopause:

- Stress can affect the hypothalamus-pituitary-ovarian axis (HPOA). The HPOA is responsible for producing hormones that regulate the menstrual cycle. If stress affects this system, it can disrupt ovulation and menstruation.

- Stress can trigger inflammation in the body, which may cause premature ovarian failure (POF). POF is when a woman stops having periods before age 40 and has stopped ovulating for at least 12 months. POF often occurs due to the surgical removal of an ovary due to cancer diagnosis or other health conditions such as endometriosis or polycystic ovary syndrome (PCOS).

- Stress can also accelerate bone density loss due to changes in hormones and increased cortisol production during times of high stress.

When you experience stress, your body produces a hormone called cortisol. This hormone increases blood sugar levels and helps you respond to environmental threats. Cortisol also triggers your body to release adrenaline—a chemical that increases heart rate and blood pressure so that you can get ready to fight or flee from danger. While these hormone changes are necessary in times of danger, when these hormones are released over some time, they can cause severe damage to your body if they remain elevated for too long.

Over time, high cortisol levels can lead to weight gain, reduced immunity, digestive problems, high blood pressure, and heart disease—all of which are known risk factors for early menopause onset or menopause difficulties. If you have been under chronic stress for an extended period, it could cause early menopause due to these effects on your body's ability to ovulate regularly

What causes stress? Stress comes from anything that

57

activates our fight-or-flight response—emotional distress, work problems, financial worries, and physical illness. Stress can also come from situations we feel powerless over (like being bullied at work) and people we feel responsible for (like children).

Here are a few stress management tips:

- Find ways to change or avoid stressful situations to lower your anxiety. For example, if sitting in traffic causes you stress, plan to take public transit or listen to an audiobook or music while you're in the car.
- Change the way you react. If something unfair or upsetting happens, choose to take a 5-minute break (outdoors, if possible) instead of getting frustrated or angry.
- Be prepared. Think of how you want to respond to challenging situations that may come up. You'll probably feel less overwhelmed.
- Pay attention to your body's feelings and signals.

- Reward yourself after you've coped with stress. Give yourself a treat, such as a bubble bath, a facial, time with a good book, or a walk in the park.

How Can I Talk With My Partner about Menopause?

It's normal to worry about talking to your partner about menopause. Talking about menopause with your partner is a great way to ensure you're both on the same page and know what to expect. However, you're not alone—many people feel afraid of talking about these issues with their partners, but it's crucial that we do! It can make a big difference in how well you and your partner understand what's happening and how well you can take care of each other through this experience.

For example, if you've been experiencing physical symptoms like hot flashes and vaginal dryness, but your partner hasn't noticed any of these things happening, they need to understand why this is happening so they can be supportive as you go through this time in your life.

It also helps if you can communicate openly about how you're feeling emotionally—what kind of mood swings you're going through or how much of an effect all these changes are having on your relationship.

It's not just about understanding what's happening physiologically—it's also about understanding what's happening psychologically and emotionally.

There are lots of ways to start the conversation:

- You could say something like, "I've been feeling really anxious lately," or "I'm having trouble sleeping at night." This is a good way to open up the conversation about what's happening for you.
- You could also try saying, "I've been thinking about how different things have felt since menopause started," which is another way of saying: I'm going through menopause, and it has made me feel differently. This might be easier for some

people than saying directly that they're going through menopause because it lets them know that their feelings are normal and expected—and gives them a chance to talk more specifically about what those feelings are like for them (e.g., "I've been feeling really anxious lately").

Here are some tips for how to talk about menopause with your partner:

1.   First and foremost, try to be understanding. Menopause is a major life change, and it's not something that many people have experienced before. You can't expect your partner to understand exactly what you're going through—but they can at least try to empathize with what you're experiencing.

2.   Start with small steps. Tell them about what's going on in your life right now (i.e., "I'm having trouble sleeping," or "I feel like my body is changing"), and ask them if they've noticed any differences in you. This way, they won't feel like they're being bombarded with information all at once—and they'll have time to process what you've told them before moving on to the

next topic!

3. Be honest about how you're feeling. Don't hold back because you think it might make your partner uncomfortable or upset them. It's important for both of you to feel comfortable talking about your experience with menopause.

Psychological Screening after Menopause

During the menopause transition, you might be more emotional than usual or feel your emotions aren't as intense as they used to be. You may also notice that your memory isn't what it used to be. Regularly checking your mental health as you transition through menopause is important.

If you start feeling like these changes are interfering with how you function in everyday life, there could be a deeper problem. It's critical to get checked out by your doctor if any of the following symptoms last for more than a month or two:

- Feeling depressed or sad all the time

- Having trouble sleeping or staying asleep at night
- Experiencing anxiety or panic attacks (feeling like you have a heart attack)
- Experiencing difficulty concentrating or remembering things that happened recently

How to Keep Yourself Psychologically Healthy

Women often experience negative emotional responses during and after menopause, such as depression and mood swings. One way to help yourself stay psychologically healthy during and after menopause is to take care of yourself. You can stay psychologically healthy during and after menopause by staying connected to your body.

Your physical health is important, but it is connected to your mind. Your body is an amazing thing, and it deserves your respect. Learning how to listen to your body, and understand its needs and limitations, will help you feel more confident and empowered. This can be done by keeping a journal where you write down how you feel daily. You can also try meditation or yoga if they appeal to you.

You can also stay psychologically healthy during and after menopause with these tips:

1. Try to stay as active as possible—This will help you fight against depression, stress, weight gain, and isolation which can be common during menopause.

2. Keep an eye on your diet—You might find that some foods make you feel better than others, so try keeping a food diary for a week or two to see if there's something you can add or cut out of your diet that will help you feel more like yourself again! At this time of your life, more than ever, you need to focus on quality foods over quantity.

3. Join a support group—This will help you feel connected to other women who are going through or have gone through similar experiences as yourself, which can be helpful when it comes to adjusting to the changes in your life as they happen!

64

4. See the doctor—If you're feeling depressed or anxious, see your doctor immediately. Some medications can help you through the early stages of menopause and keep your moods stable.

5. Reduce stress—Consider ways that you can reduce stress in your life. Is there anything weighing on your mind? Are any issues at work or home that need to be addressed? If so, make time for dealing with them—don't let them pile up!

6. Be kind to yourself— You're going through a lot right now, and it's okay if you don't get it right every time. It's also okay if you don't feel like trying at all some days! Remember that this is just a phase. You will come out on the other side and be better than ever because of it!

7. Find what works for you—What works for one person might not work for another, so try different things until something clicks! Maybe try meditating or exercising more? Maybe talk with your friends about their experiences with menopause. Whatever it is, don't forget about yourself just because you're busy taking care of others!

8. *Take care of yourself first*—Take care of everyone else around you second (and only if there's still time). This isn't selfish. Self-care is vital because if we don't take care of ourselves first, how can we expect anyone else to do so?

CHAPTER 3: THE BODY

Hormones

Hormones are chemical messengers that travel through our bloodstream and tell other body parts what to do. Hormones control how we feel and how we behave. Some of the most important hormones in our bodies are the reproductive or sex hormones. They control reproductive functions like puberty, fertility, sexual desire, and other characteristics related to gender identities, like facial hair growth or breast growth during puberty for males versus females, respectively. They also play essential roles in other areas, such as metabolism (how fast we burn calories),

67

muscle gain/loss (muscle-building exercises such as lifting weights or running), and mood swings (anxiety or depression).

The key reproductive hormones

The key reproductive hormones are

- Estrogen
- Progesterone
- Testosterone

Estrogen

Estrogen is a sex hormone responsible for female sexual characteristics. It is produced in the ovaries and adrenal glands. Estrogen is the hormone that controls your menstrual cycle, regulates your reproductive organs, and helps to maintain your bone density and guard against osteoporosis. Estrogen is vital for the development of the female reproductive system during puberty. It also plays a role in regulating the menstrual cycle and ovulation. Estrogen helps maintain the elasticity of blood vessels and contributes to normal blood clotting.

Estrogen levels fluctuate throughout your lifetime. They are higher before puberty, lower during menopause, and increase again during perimenopause (the time leading up to menopause).

- Estrogen Dominance

Estrogen dominance is a condition caused by an imbalance (estrogen too high) in your body's estrogen levels. It is characterized by water retention, mood swings and migraines, weight gain, bloating, and breast tenderness. The most common cause of estrogen dominance is an imbalance between the level of estrogen produced by your body and the level of progesterone. When these hormones are out of balance, it can lead to many health problems, including breast cancer.

If you have any of the symptoms listed above, talk to your doctor about testosterone replacement therapy (TRT). TRT has been shown to help restore balance in your hormone levels which can alleviate many symptoms associated with estrogen dominance and other hormonal imbalances.

Progesterone

Progesterone is also a sex hormone, but it's produced by the corpus luteum of the ovaries after an egg has been released during ovulation—it prepares a woman's uterus for pregnancy by thickening its lining.

Testosterone

Testosterone, which is also produced by the ovaries (in addition to male testes), is responsible for developing secondary sex characteristics such as body hair and muscle mass; it's also responsible for maintaining bone density during puberty. Testosterone is produced in both men and women and plays a role in sexual development and functioning, including libido and sperm production.

Hormonal imbalance

Hormonal imbalance is a condition in which the levels of hormones such as estrogen and progesterone are not in the correct ratios. Hormonal imbalance can cause symptoms such as irregular periods, abnormal vaginal discharge, or headaches.

The female body undergoes many hormonal changes throughout life. The first change occurs when a girl begins puberty (usually between nine and 13). This change occurs because of the increase in estrogen levels. Estrogen causes breast development and body hair growth in girls. It also causes the uterus to begin growing its lining for pregnancy.

Another hormone change occurs during pregnancy when an increase in progesterone levels prepares the uterus for pregnancy. After childbirth, there is another change in hormone levels as they decrease back down to normal levels.

There are many other causes of hormonal imbalance, including:

- Ovarian tumors or cysts
- Pelvic inflammatory disease
- Endometriosis
- Adrenal gland disorders

The most common causes of hormonal imbalance

include:

- Polycystic ovarian syndrome (PCOS)
- Menopause

Hormones and Menopause

During menopause, your body goes through some significant hormone changes. The biggest ones are in the estrogen and progesterone levels.

Going through menopause, you might notice that these hormones are no longer being produced in their usual amounts. This can cause many symptoms, such as hot flashes, night sweats, vaginal dryness (which can lead to painful sex), and irregular periods. It's important to talk with your doctor if these symptoms are bothering you so they can help prescribe treatment options that work best for you!

As you get older, your body will begin to make less and less estrogen—and it could cause bone loss and memory loss issues. When this happens, you may be prescribed hormone replacement therapy (HRT) to help maintain balance. The good news is that there are many healthy ways to manage the symptoms of menopause without using HRT or experiencing side effects from synthetic hormones!

<u>Sex and Sexuality</u>

Our sexuality is tied to many aspects of our life, including our emotional, physical, and social well-being. It's normal to feel worried about how menopause will affect your sex life. You might wonder if you'll be able to have sex at all anymore or if it will be different than it was before menopause started. But don't worry! Your sex life doesn't have to change as much as you think.

You might become more sensitive during sex after menopause because there are fewer hormones in your body, which means less lubrication. This can make penetration painful or difficult and reduce your desire for sex. That's why it's important to use lubricant when you have sex after menopause.

Some women find they're less interested in sex after menopause because they don't feel like having an orgasm anymore—and that's totally normal! Your

73

partner may also find that his erection becomes weaker and that he takes longer to reach orgasm due to his own hormonal changes, such as decreased testosterone levels.

You may also experience changes in your body image and self-esteem as you go through menopause, which can impact your ability to enjoy sex. You may feel less attractive physically, and this may lead to a decrease in sexual desire. The effects that menopause will have on your sex life largely depend on how long you've been dealing with menopause symptoms. If you're still in the early stages, when your hormone levels are still fluctuating, and you're only just starting to experience hot flashes, then it's likely that the changes in your body won't be too drastic. This means that the sex drive might not change much at all—after all, there's nothing like a bit of heat to get you in the mood!

However, if you're further along in menopause and experiencing more severe symptoms such as hot flashes and vaginal dryness, these issues could affect your sex life. Hot flashes can be distracting during foreplay and intercourse, while vaginal dryness may cause pain during penetration or make intercourse uncomfortable for both partners.

Of course, this doesn't mean you should stop having sex once you hit menopause. It just means that it's important to talk with your partner about any changes (or lack thereof) so they can help support you!

There are many ways to overcome these problems. Many hormone-replacement therapies (HRT) can help alleviate some of these symptoms by restoring natural estrogen, progesterone, and testosterone levels. It is important to remember that not all women experience the same symptoms during menopause, so it is important to talk with your doctor about what medications are right for you.

Will I lose desire?

Your sexual desire depends on many factors besides your hormone levels, including your emotional makeup, physical health, and social and cultural background. During menopause, your sex hormone levels gradually decrease. Your sexual desire and arousal from sexual stimulation may also decrease.

Your desire can also be affected if having intercourse becomes painful or if you're bothered by menopausal symptoms, such as hot flashes, vaginal dryness, insomnia, or irritability.

Do I still need to practice safe sex after menopause?

The short answer is yes; you still need to practice safe sex after menopause.

While it's true that your risk of pregnancy is lower after menopause than before, that doesn't mean you should stop using protection altogether. It is still possible to contract sexually transmitted diseases (STDs), including HIV/AIDS.

Now that you're older and have a higher chance of having other health issues (like heart disease or diabetes), it's even more important to protect yourself against STDs. If you have an STD, it might be hard for your body to fight off other illnesses or develop serious complications.

Will I enjoy sex as I get older?

The whole issue of sexuality as we age is significant for both men and women. Sex and sexuality do change as we age. The human body tends to respond differently – for most people, the response is slower, less intense, but not less enjoyable with age. However, men and women are both capable of sexual response until they die.

Sexual activity can be a pleasurable and healthy experience for any woman regardless of age, stage of life, or physical abilities. The choice to abstain from sex is also normal and healthy.

How can I improve my sexual health after menopause?

Here are some simple things you can do:

- Eat a balanced diet with plenty of fruits and vegetables.
- Exercise regularly, at least three times per week, for 30 minutes or more each time.
- Reduce stress by meditating, taking a bath, or going for walks in nature.

- Reduce alcohol consumption to one drink per day (if you're drinking).
- Keep up with your regular doctor visits.
- Make sure there is mutual respect between you and your partner.
- Talk to your partner about the changes in your body and how they can help you feel more comfortable.
- Spend more time in foreplay. Learn about your body and what makes you feel sexually excited, and communicate this to your partner.
- Don't be afraid to address discomfort. To ensure sex is pleasurable for both of you, it is essential to address any discomfort immediately. Vaginal pain and dryness are common symptoms in menopausal women and can lead to uncomfortable or painful sex. Use lubricants.
- Try new methods of intimacy. There are various ways to have a strong intimate relationship without penetrative sex. This is especially helpful if you're experiencing a mind-body disconnect, where you want to

have sex even though your body might not cooperate. Examples include:

- o Oral sex
- o Explicit games or conversation
- o Erotic massage
- o Erotic books and videos

- Don't give up on sex. Instead of waiting until you feel desire, let yourself be willing. You may not start out "in the mood," but most women can get in the mood given enough time and foreplay.

- Explore treatment options. Reach out to your healthcare provider to discuss potential treatment options to help make sex more enjoyable for you and your partner.

Benefits of sex

- Sex helps to relieve stress.
- Sex boosts your immune system.
- Sex burns fat and increases blood flow in your body.
- Sex strengthens your pelvic muscles and reduces incontinence later in life.

- People who have sex often have higher levels of naturally produced sex hormones, which help to stimulate sexual desire.
- Sex can increase your self-esteem.
- Sex enhances feelings of intimacy with your partner.

Maintaining Sexual Health

Maintaining sexual health requires attention and a little effort. You should stay informed about safe choices, healthy behaviors, and how your body works. By educating yourself and listening to your body, you don't have to let menopause be the end of your sex life. By making a few minor changes and staying on top of your sexual health, you can continue having great sex no matter your age.

Body Changes

Weight

Does your weight seem to be creeping up, even though you're not eating more or exercising less? You may be experiencing menopause.

Weight gain is one of the most common side effects of menopause. It is estimated that between 20% and 40% of women experience weight gain after menopause. This is due to changes in hormones during the female reproductive cycle. In particular, estrogen levels drop after menopause which can cause fat deposits to increase around the waistline.

Many factors contribute to this, including:

- Decrease in energy
- Increase in appetite
- Loss of muscle mass
- Hormone changes lead to less thyroid hormone production, which helps regulate metabolism

However, there are several things you can do to help prevent weight gain during this time:

1) Eat a healthy diet - include plenty of fruits, vegetables, whole grains, and lean meats like chicken or fish. Make every calorie count and go for quality rather than quantity.

2) Exercise regularly - regular physical activity will help keep your metabolism high which will help prevent weight gain when combined with eating healthy foods.

3) Get adequate sleep - getting enough sleep each night will help regulate hormone levels so they don't fluctuate as much throughout the day.

Hot Flashes

Do you ever feel like you're a walking, talking space heater?

If so, you're not alone! Hot flashes are one of the most common symptoms of menopause. They're also one of the most annoying because they can make it difficult to do just about anything and make you feel like your body is out of control.

But never fear—we're here to help!

What Are Hot Flashes?

Hot flashes are when your body overheats in response to hormonal changes that occur during menopause (or

82

other hormone changes). The temperature in your body gets too high, causing you to sweat profusely and feel like you're overheating from the inside out—even if the room isn't overly warm. When this happens, it's called having a hot flash.

What Causes Hot Flashes?

Hot flashes happen because of an imbalance between estrogen (the hormone that makes women act like women) and progesterone (the hormone responsible for making us feel calm). During menopause, our bodies stop producing enough progesterone, which causes our bodies' temperatures to elevate. Hot flashes happen when your body gets too hot, and your brain responds by sending signals to cool down. These signals can cause tingling, flushing, sweating, and rapid heartbeat, which are unpleasant and sometimes even embarrassing.

How to stop Hot Flashes

The good news is that hot flashes are temporary. You'll probably start noticing them about two years before menopause starts, and they'll probably go away after about six months. If they're affecting your quality of life or making you feel uncomfortable, there are ways to reduce them!

Here are some tips:

- **Keep plenty of cold water around** -- this will help decrease your core temperature and keep you hydrated at the same time! It also helps flush out toxins from your body.
- **Avoid alcohol and caffeine** -- both of these things can make your heart beat faster and cause hot flashes in some people.
- **Exercise regularly** improves circulation throughout the body, which means more oxygen gets where it needs to.
- **Keep stress under control** by practicing mindfulness or meditation exercises or even just taking some time each day to sit quietly without distractions (like phones or computers) to clear your mind.

- **Try natural remedies** like ginger tea (add a little honey for sweetness) or lemon balm tea.
- **Adopt a healthy lifestyle** with regular exercise, good sleep habits, and a balanced diet filled with fruits and vegetables.

If these interventions aren't working for you, talk with your doctor about other treatment options, such as hormone replacement therapy (HRT). HRT is a mostly safe and effective way to manage hot flashes caused by menopause; however, it should only be used under medical supervision since it could increase your risk of breast cancer if used without proper follow-up care.

Vaginal Dryness

Vaginal dryness after menopause is a common issue affecting women's sex lives. While it can be a sign of a medical problem, including vaginal atrophy, it's usually a normal issue that can be addressed with lifestyle changes and medication.

How to treat

Many natural herbal remedies can help alleviate this problem, and we're here to tell you how to find the best one for you.

The first step is to ensure you're drinking enough water daily. Water helps keep your body hydrated and healthy, and it also helps keep your vaginal tissues moist and supple. If you're dehydrated, drinking more water will go a long way toward keeping your vaginal tissues moisturized.

Next, try taking a probiotic supplement each day. Probiotics are beneficial bacteria that live in your digestive tract, improving digestion and helping to ward off harmful bacteria and viruses. They can also help balance the pH of your vagina. If it's imbalanced, it may contribute to dryness or itching.

Finally, suppose these steps don't work for you. In that case, it's time to see a doctor about prescription vaginal moisturizers like Replens or Vagifem, which contain estrogen that helps restore moisture levels in the vagina and reduce inflammation.

Here are some additional tips:

- Try using a water-based lubricant like Astroglide or KY Jelly. These can be found at most drug stores.
- Use a suitable moisturizing cream or lotion on your vagina before having sex. You can find these products at most drugstores. Avoid perfumed ones.
- Consider talking with your doctor about taking hormone replacement therapy (HRT). This treatment is usually prescribed by a gynecologist or endocrinologist specializing in women's health issues.
- Kegel exercises (pelvic floor muscle exercises) - Kegel exercises for your pelvic floor muscles can help relieve and prevent some vaginal and bladder symptoms caused by low muscle tone. Doing Kegels regularly can also help increase your enjoyment of sexual intimacy.

Skin, Hair, and Nails

Menopause can be tough for your skin, nails, and hair. You might notice that your skin gets drier or more oily than usual. Or maybe you see new fine lines. It's not just your imagination—menopause causes a change in hormone levels that affect how your body functions, including how easily it absorbs nutrients and holds on to water.

Here are some ways to support menopausal skin:

1. Try a weekly face mask with hyaluronic acid— it helps skin look plump and hydrated by drawing in moisture.
2. Use products containing retinol or peptides to smooth out wrinkles.
3. Moisturize with products that contain ceramides to help seal in moisture and protect against dryness.
4. Use exfoliating scrubs to remove dead skin cells (which can clog pores).
5. Eat a healthy diet with plenty of fruits and vegetables, whole grains, lean proteins, and healthy fats such as olive oil, avocados, and nuts.
6. Drink lots of water! Hydration is key for healthy skin.

7. Take an omega-3 supplement or eat more salmon or other fatty fish that contains omega-3s every week or two (or as often as you'd like). These nutrients help keep your skin soft and supple and reduce inflammation in your body overall!

8. Use a moisturizer with SPF 15 every day—and even more frequently if you spend time outside during daylight hours (which helps reduce wrinkles). Remember, sunscreen isn't just for summer! You should wear it year-round to protect yourself from sun damage that can lead to cancer later in life.

CHAPTER 4: HORMONE REPLACEMENT THERAPY (HRT)

While we've mentioned HRT in previous chapters, we will look at it more in-depth in this chapter. Hormone replacement therapy (HRT) is a common treatment for low or imbalanced hormone levels. It's also used to treat symptoms of menopause and other conditions. However, HRT has been surrounded by controversy since it was first developed, and myths and questions about its safety still exist today.

The Myths and Mystery of HRT

Have you asked your doctor about hormone

replacement therapy? If not, maybe you should.

HRT is a clinical treatment for menopause symptoms that has been shown to relieve hot flashes, night sweats, vaginal dryness, and urinary incontinence. It can also help slow bone loss in women who have gone through menopause. There's no denying that HRT is an effective treatment for the symptoms of menopause—but there are some myths surrounding this treatment that may be keeping you from asking your doctor about it.

Let's take a look at some of the most common myths out there and see how they stack up with the facts:

Myth 1: HRT is only for older women—and therefore not right for me. This is one of the most common myths about hormone replacement therapy! Younger women can also benefit from HRT if they experience severe hot flashes or other symptoms associated with menopause. The key is finding a dosage that works best for your body type and lifestyle needs so that you feel comfortable taking it regularly.

Myth 2: HRT causes cancer and heart disease. This isn't necessarily true—it might reduce your risk of these diseases.

Myth 3: HRT causes osteoporosis or other bone-related problems. Some people believe that taking hormones causes people to lose bone density, which leads to osteoporosis later in life. However, this is not true! Women who take hormones have higher bone density than those who don't take them—they're 30% less likely to suffer from hip fractures or other bone-related problems than those who don't take hormones.

Many people think that because it contains estrogen (which has been linked to breast cancer), HRT must be bad for you. Studies have shown that this isn't true. The truth is that HRT is safe for most women.

HRT can also help prevent heart disease by lowering LDL cholesterol levels (the bad kind) while raising HDL cholesterol levels (the good kind). This can help reduce your risk of stroke by nearly half!

Types of HRT

There are two types of HRT: "systemic" and "local."

Systemic HRT

Hormones are released into your bloodstream. They affect the organs and tissues throughout the body to help relieve a range of menopausal symptoms, such as hot flashes. This type of HRT is available in many forms, including pills, skin patches, creams, and sprays. If progesterone (progestin) is also prescribed, it can be given alone or combined with estrogen in one prescription.

Local HRT

Hormones are applied directly to certain areas of the body, such as the vagina. They can relieve specific menopausal symptoms, including vaginal dryness, pain during sex, and bladder problems. Local HRT is available in creams, tablets, and rings. Vaginal estrogen can usually be used safely, but women who've had breast cancer or blood clots need to talk with their doctor before using any form of estrogen.

Benefits of HRT

Hormone therapy is a common treatment for women who have had a hysterectomy or who are going through menopause. It can also treat other conditions, such as endometriosis, polycystic ovary syndrome (PCOS), and breast cancer.

Hormone therapy may help to:

- Improve your mood
- Reduce irregular bleeding
- Relieve vaginal dryness and soreness
- Reduce the frequency and severity of hot flashes and night sweats
- Improve sleep problems
- Slow the loss of skin collagen, which enables skin and muscle to stretch
- Reduce the risk of developing osteoporosis
- Reduce the risk of cardiovascular disease

In addition, hormone therapy may improve your quality of life by reducing the impact of menopause on your daily life.

Risks and Side Effects of HRT

HRT risks relate to each woman's age, when HRT is started during the menopause transition, and how long HRT is taken. Short-term use in early menopause is generally less risky than starting HRT later in menopause.

The most common risk is blood clots, which can be fatal. This is why taking hormones for the first time should always be done under medical supervision. Other risks include high blood pressure, high cholesterol, cancer, and diabetes. These conditions can lead to heart disease and other serious health issues. Women who take hormones should have regular check-ups with their doctor to monitor their overall health.

Side effects from HRT are uncommon but might include:

- Irregular vaginal bleeding
- Swollen or tender breasts
- Headaches, nausea, or bloating

- Leg cramps
- Vaginal discharge

Making a Decision about HRT

Every woman is unique. Only you know how severe or distressing your menopause symptoms are. In making your decision, consider both your quality of life and the potential risks of HRT.

Discuss your specific risks and benefits with your doctor or other care practitioners. You can also discuss additional options for managing your symptoms. Learn as much as you can about your choices before starting HRT.

Hormone therapy needs to be individualized to meet each woman's needs. If you decide on HRT, tell your doctor about your symptoms and health status at every appointment. HRT doses can be adjusted or stopped as needed.

CHAPTER 5: TAKING BACK CONTROL

It's important to think about menopause and plan to experience this critical transition positively because it is a time when you can change your life for the better. Menopause marks the beginning of a new chapter in your life, and it's up to you to ensure it's a good one.

Many women fear menopause because they don't know what will happen or how to cope with it. But there are so many ways to help yourself through this transition! You can start by learning all about it: what happens physically and emotionally, how long it takes and why, etc. Then you can decide whether or not you

99

want to use hormones (and if so, which ones). Once you have all the information, choose an approach that makes sense for YOU!

Menopause can be an exhilarating time in your life! Don't let it be something that just happens to you but rather something that you manage and take control of. We know that the healthier and fitter you are, the less chance there is of having a difficult time when going through menopause. So diet, exercise, and lifestyle are significant factors, and the younger you start getting yourself ready, the better!

Planning and Reflection

Thinking about how you plan to experience this critical transition positively is essential because you want to feel good and be prepared for what's to come. You don't want to feel like your body is betraying you or that it's not working the way it should. You want to be able to focus on your life and the things that are important to you rather than being distracted by symptoms that might be making it difficult for you to do so.

You also don't want your friends, family members, or coworkers feeling awkward around you because they don't know what to say or do when they see your symptoms in action—and we all know how awkward an uncomfortable silence can be!

Think about menopause like you would any other important transition in your life. For example, if you were moving to a new city or starting a new job, you might take some time to plan ahead and make sure that the move goes smoothly. You might also want to consider whether there are any special considerations for the people around you—for example, if you're moving away from family and friends, how can you make sure they know how to contact you?

The same goes for menopause. The best way to make sure that this transition goes smoothly is to think about it in advance and make a plan for how to experience it positively. You can work with your doctor or nurse practitioner to determine when menopause will start and ensure that your lifestyle choices align with those changes.

Menopause is an important transition that can be experienced in a positive, healthy way. Many women experience menopause as an opportunity to re-evaluate their lives and start new projects they've always wanted to do. It is also a time when many women find themselves more connected with their emotions and their spirituality than ever before.

It's important to plan and reflect on what you want to do to make the most of this time in your life.

Think about what you want from this transition.

Do you want to continue working?

Are there any health conditions that you need to manage?

What is your support system like?

How are you feeling right now?

Once you've reflected on these questions, start making a plan! This is an excellent opportunity to reflect on your life and decide what you want it to look like in the future. Maybe you'll want to take some time off work, or perhaps you'll want to talk with your boss about working remotely. Maybe you'll want to take some time for yourself—whatever it is, make sure your needs are prioritized. You might decide that you want to travel or volunteer more. Whatever it is, now is the time to think about what's important to you and plan to have an amazing experience during this time of transition.

How to Stay Healthy During Menopause

Menopause is a time of significant change and adjustment, but it doesn't have to mean drastic lifestyle changes. Here are some ways you can make positive lifestyle changes that will help you stay healthy during menopause:

1. Make sure you're getting enough calcium
Calcium is an integral part of bone health, and it's crucial in women going through menopause. Women generally lose up to 10% of bone mass in the first five years after menopause. If you aren't getting enough

calcium, your bones may become brittle and prone to fractures. Getting enough calcium can help prevent this from happening!

Aim for a dietary calcium intake of around 1300mg per day. This is found in three to four dairy serves. If you prefer non-dairy calcium sources, they include hard tofu, almonds, Brazil nuts, tahini, dark green leafy vegetables, and fish with bones, such as canned sardines.

Remember that vitamin D helps with calcium absorption, so ensure you get enough sunshine.

2. Eat more fruits and vegetables

Fruits and vegetables are a great source of vitamins and minerals that can help keep your body running smoothly as it adjusts to its new state of balance. Add extra servings of fruit or vegetables into your daily diet to ensure you get all the nutrients you need!

3. Exercise regularly

Exercise has been shown to help with many different aspects of health throughout life—including during menopause—so it's important not to neglect this aspect of wellness when making lifestyle changes! Try fitting in 30 minutes or more of exercise every day (or break it up into smaller chunks), and make sure it includes stretching.

4. Stay hydrated

Drink plenty of water throughout the day. It helps flush toxins from your body and keeps your kidneys healthy.

5. Manage your stress levels

Stress is another common symptom during menopause because it affects hormone levels, leading to mood swings or anxiety attacks if left unmanaged properly! One way we've found helpful is through meditation—try taking time out each day just for yourself to relax by focusing on something calm like nature or listening to music while doing deep breathing exercises every morning before work, so it becomes routine.

6. Talk

Talking about these feelings with friends and family is

important so they can help you through them. You may also want to see a therapist or counselor who specializes in working with women going through menopause so they can give you tips on how best to deal with those issues, as well as any others that come up at this time (such as sleep problems).

Sleep

Sleep is a necessary part of life, but it becomes increasingly difficult as we age. Sleep is essential for the body to function well, especially as we age. Many things, such as menopause, medications, and depression, can affect sleep. Menopause can be one of the most challenging times in a woman's life due to hot flashes and night sweats. This can make it very hard for them to get quality sleep at night without waking up feeling tired every morning.

You may wake up more frequently throughout the night or feel groggy in the morning when you don't get enough sleep. A lack of sleep can also lead to memory loss or mood swings, making it difficult for you to cope with the symptoms associated with menopause.

In addition to these physical symptoms, many women report having trouble falling asleep at night and staying asleep. It is reported that this could be due to increased cortisol levels (a stress hormone) during menopause.

How to improve your sleep

These symptoms are normal, but if they interfere with your daily life, you should talk to your doctor about what might be causing them. They can help determine if any other underlying issues need attention.

In addition to consulting with your doctor, there are some steps you can take on your own to improve your sleep quality during this time in your life:

- Avoid caffeine after noon (and limit your intake throughout the day)
- Take walks outside during daylight hours
- Try different sleeping positions; for example, lying on your left side may make it easier for you to fall asleep
- Don't eat heavy foods late at night

- Get up at the same time every day, even if you don't feel tired

- Exercise regularly but avoid vigorous exercise close to bedtime

- Try relaxation exercises before bedtime—deep breathing is a great way to relax your muscles and mind before bed so that both are ready for rest.

- Keep your bedroom cool at night, and ensure you have a comfortable mattress that doesn't cause back pain or stiffness. You should also consider buying a new pillow if yours isn't supportive enough.

- Make sure there aren't any distractions in the bedroom, like TVs or computers, that might keep you up at night. You should also remove any clutter from the room so it doesn't distract you from falling asleep quickly when bedtime comes around each night. In short, make your bedroom a quiet haven.

- Keeping a consistent sleep schedule is key to getting enough rest each night. Try going to bed and waking up at the same time each day, including on weekends. This will help your body adjust to a regular sleep schedule and make it easier to fall asleep at night.

- Create a relaxing bedtime routine. This can help you wind down after a busy day and prepare your body for sleep. Some ideas include taking a bath or shower, reading a book or magazine, meditating or practicing deep breathing exercises, listening to soothing music, or having sex with your partner (if they're willing).

Exercise

When you're in menopause, it can be hard to motivate yourself to get moving. But physical activity is important for your overall health and can help ease some of the symptoms of menopause.

Exercise can:

- Help relieve the symptoms associated with menopause, such as hot flashes and night sweats

- Boost your mood and lessen stress, which hormonal changes during menopause can cause
- Reduce your risk of heart disease, diabetes, and osteoporosis
- Reduce your risk of breast cancer

When you exercise, especially if you do strength-training exercises like squats or deadlifts, your body releases more estrogen and progesterone, which helps with hot flashes and sleep problems that can come with menopause. Now that you know that exercise helps with menopause symptoms, here are some tips on how to start exercising!

1) Start slowly. Don't try to go from sitting on the couch watching Netflix all day to running a marathon—it won't work out well for anybody! Start by walking at a brisk pace for 30 minutes three times per week. Once you are into a routine and feel comfortable with this, increase it to five times a week. Vary your route to keep it interesting, or walk with a friend.

2) Find an activity that works for you. If running isn't your thing, but weightlifting is what gets you going, then go for it! The key is finding something that gives you energy instead of taking it away. You are more likely to stick with an activity you enjoy.

3) Exercise examples to explore: Exercising can be done in various ways, but the main thing is to get moving. Try walking, swimming, yoga and pilates classes, weight training, and resistance training are just a few examples. Cycling or dancing may be more of your thing. The important thing is to find something that works for you!

Diet

What you eat will have a significant impact on your health. Good nutrition supports your hormonal health, energy levels, and mood by providing the nutrients your body needs to function at its best. Not only does this help you feel empowered and energized throughout the day, but it also contributes to your overall health and wellness.

You should first know that your body requires certain vitamins and minerals to produce certain hormones. For example, vitamin B6 is necessary for the proper production of serotonin—the "happy hormone"—while zinc is essential for testosterone production. If you don't get enough of these nutrients from your diet, it can impact how well you feel physically and emotionally.

Your body also needs certain fats and proteins to produce optimal amounts of estrogen, progesterone, and testosterone. These three key hormones regulate most of our reproductive functions and other essential functions like bone density or blood pressure levels. If you don't consume enough fat or protein, this can result in decreased hormone production, which may cause symptoms like headaches or PMS symptoms like bloating or breast tenderness during each month's menstruation cycles!

Healthy Diet and Hormonal Health

Many factors, including diet, determine hormonal health. When we eat foods high in sugar and refined carbs, our bodies release insulin to help store those carbohydrates as fat. This causes blood sugar levels to spike and crash—a pattern that can lead to mood swings, fatigue, and even depression. It doesn't have to be that way! A healthy diet can help keep your hormones balanced and support optimal energy levels. The key is eating whole foods like fruits and vegetables that give you the nutrients your body needs without causing spikes in blood sugar or inflammation (which can lead to weight gain).

Energy and Vitality

You want to focus on the things that are important to you. You want to have the energy and vitality to do those things. But how do you get the energy and vitality you need?

You already know that eating healthy foods is key to maintaining a healthy lifestyle and losing weight, but did you know that certain foods can help you focus better? There are many different ways to get these nutrients into your diet.

A good start is incorporating foods high in omega-3 fatty acids into your diet. These include salmon, sardines, walnuts, flax seed oil, and chia seeds. Omega-3 fatty acids help keep your brain cells healthy by increasing circulation and improving blood flow to

113

the brain. They also increase memory function and improve mood by reducing inflammation throughout the body.

It would be best to consider adding foods rich in vitamin D into your diet. It's an essential vitamin for strong bones and teeth but also helps regulate moods by controlling serotonin levels in the body (which creates feelings of happiness). Vitamin D can be found in fortified milk products and fish such as tuna or salmon if consumed regularly over time.

What food to eat and avoid

Here's a quick rundown of what foods to eat and avoid during menopause.

What to eat

A diet that contains some healthy fats and is high in fiber can help reduce vaginal dryness or irritation and decrease pain during intercourse, which are both common symptoms of menopause. Foods containing fat-soluble vitamin E—such as nuts, seeds, avocado, and olive oil—are also good for vaginal health because they have antioxidant properties that protect against free radicals (which cause inflammation).

It is also known that calcium may help reduce hot flashes by preventing the release of estrogen from bone tissue. Calcium-rich foods include milk (2% or higher), yogurt (plain), and cheese (the low-fat kind).

- Low-fat dairy products like yogurt and cheese can help reduce hot flashes.
- Whole grains, such as whole grain bread and cereals, are digested slowly to help regulate your insulin levels so they don't fluctuate wildly during the day. This can reduce the severity of other menopausal symptoms like mood swings or depression.
- Fruits and vegetables contain antioxidants that protect against cell damage caused by free radicals—and since cells are damaged every day in your body (especially when you're going through menopause), these foods are essential during this time!

Here are some common symptoms and how certain nutrients might help relieve them:

- Hot flashes

Vitamin B6 helps regulate estrogen levels in the body and reduce hot flashes; magnesium has also been shown to decrease hot flashes by increasing blood flow to the skin (which cools it off). To help keep your body healthy during menopause, eat foods rich in phytoestrogens, which can help reduce hot flashes and other menopausal symptoms. Phytoestrogens are plant chemicals that mimic the effects of estrogen. Foods high in phytoestrogens include soybeans, flaxseeds, some beans, sesame seeds, and whole grains.

- Vaginal dryness

Vitamin E helps keep cells healthy and moist; omega-3 oils also keep tissues moisturized and flexible. Good sources of vitamin E include seed oils, almonds, peanuts, and avocados. Oily fish, flaxseeds, and chia seeds are good sources of omega-3s.

- Mood swings

Omega-3 fats help balance moods by reducing inflammation in the brain; vitamin E improves memory function, which helps reduce stress

What to avoid

Saturated fats from red meat and whole milk dairy products raise bad cholesterol levels, increasing your risk of heart disease. However, it is suggested that eating moderate amounts of fatty fish may improve your heart's health! You should also avoid foods that may cause inflammation in your body. These include saturated fats, trans fats, and refined carbohydrates like white bread and white rice. Go easy on salt and sodium. Eating too much sodium may cause loss of calcium via urination and can increase your blood pressure.

While knowing what to eat and what to avoid may seem confusing, some basic good nutrition principles will help. Try to eat primarily plant-based whole foods. This includes a selection of fruit, vegetables, nuts, seeds, and legumes. Add a small amount of healthy oils such as olive oil, nut butters, and avocados. If you're not vegan or vegetarian, add low-fat dairy, lean meat, and fish. Avoid refined foods such as white bread and sugary treats.

<u>Herbs</u>

Herbs can help reduce the symptoms of menopause by balancing hormones and helping reduce stress levels. Some herbs have hormone-balancing properties, while others promote relaxation or increase circulation. Herbs such as black cohosh, dong Quai, wild yam root, and licorice root have been used for centuries to treat hormonal imbalances during menopause. These herbs are known as phytoestrogens because they mimic estrogen in the body without causing side effects like synthetic hormone replacement therapy does.

Herbs can also be used during menopause as an alternative HRT. HRT has been shown to increase the risk of breast cancer and heart disease in some women, so herbal supplements may be a better option for those who would rather not take synthetic hormones or drugs linked to these side effects.

Here are some herbs that can help.

Black cohosh

This herb has been shown to help reduce hot flashes and other symptoms of menopause.

Red raspberry leaf

This herb helps with menstrual cramps, which often become worse during perimenopause.

Stinging nettle

This herb helps your body produce more estrogen, lowering hot flashes and other symptoms of menopause.

Chaste tree berry

This herb, also known as Vitex, has been shown to reduce hot flashes, night sweats, and other menopause-related symptoms by up to 40%. It's considered safe to take long-term and doesn't interact with any medications currently on the market.

Red clover

Red clover has been shown in some studies to be effective at reducing hot flashes, night sweats, vaginal dryness, and mood swings associated with menopause. However, more research is needed before we can definitively say whether red clover works effectively for these purposes.

Ginseng

Ginseng is often used as an alternative therapy in cases where patients don't desire HRT. It helps regulate blood sugar levels and improves sleep quality while reducing anxiety levels.

Dong Quai

Dong Quai is another herb that can be used as a natural alternative to HRT by regulating blood sugar levels while reducing anxiety levels and improving sleep quality (although it may not work as well for menopausal women experiencing severe hot flashes).

Supplements

If you're looking for a safe and natural way to help manage menopause symptoms, consider supplements. These preparations can be an excellent way to supplement your diet with vitamins and minerals.

They can also provide a higher dose of nutrients than what is typically found in food alone.

Many different types of supplements are available for menopause symptoms, including:

Calcium

Calcium supplements can help improve bone density, which may reduce the risk of osteoporosis. Calcium also helps prevent hot flashes and night sweats by relaxing blood vessels near the skin's surface. Calcium is crucial for managing mood swings during menopause (and beyond).

Collagen

Every woman over 40 should be taking a collagen supplement. Collagen is the most abundant protein in the body and can be found in the skin, tendons, ligaments, and bones. As we age, our bodies produce less collagen; over time, this causes our skin to sag, wrinkles to appear, and our joints to become stiffer.

The good news is that collagen supplements are an easy way to combat these changes.

121

Collagen supplements are made from the same type of protein found in the body. When taken orally, it can help repair damaged tissue by encouraging new collagen production.

The natural aging process can take a toll on your skin, joints, and bones. Collagen helps strengthen your bones by providing the nutrients needed to rebuild themselves after injury or stress. It also helps improve skin elasticity, giving it a more youthful appearance by slowing down the rate at which your skin loses moisture. This helps keep fine lines around your eyes and mouth under control, so you don't need Botox injections as often! Taking collagen supplements can reduce joint pain from conditions like arthritis by up to 50%.

Vitamin E

Vitamin E has been shown to relieve hot flashes and night sweats by reducing inflammation throughout your body. It also supports heart health by helping clear arteries of plaque build-up, which can cause heart disease.

Vitamin A

This vitamin is crucial for healthy skin and bones, but it's also important for reproductive health. It helps maintain the function of the ovaries and testes, which are affected during menopause.

Vitamin D3

Vitamin D3 helps regulate hormones in the body and prevent bone loss. It is reported that women who take Vitamin D have lower rates of menopausal symptoms. You can find Vitamin D3 in most grocery stores and health food stores.

Omega-3 fatty acids

Omega-3 fatty acids have been shown to affect mood and heart health positively. They also help with symptoms of menopause, including hot flashes, night sweats, fatigue, and depression. The American Heart Association recommends eating two 3.5-ounce servings of fatty fish a week because of the health benefits of the omega-3 fatty acids DHA (docosahexaenoic acid) and EPA (eicosapentaenoic acid).

Maca

Maca provides general symptom relief, especially for hot flashes, night sweats, and

mood.

Melatonin

Our brains naturally produce this hormone in response to darkness. Melatonin helps those with insomnia and other sleep disorders to fall asleep. One to three milligrams taken two hours before bedtime is recommended for those with sleep problems.

Essential Oil and Aromatherapy

One way to cope with menopause's irritating symptoms, like anxiety and sleep problems, is through aromatherapy, which uses fragrances to help bring on feelings of relaxation, calmness, and ease. Essential oils are a great place to start when looking for aromatherapy products for menopause, as they're usually made with all-natural ingredients and provide safe and effective results.

124

Essential oils are extracted from herbs or flowers using cold-pressing or steam distillation. This process preserves their natural properties—including the therapeutic benefits—without adding anything else into the mix. They're also very concentrated: a single drop can have as much aroma as an entire cup of tea!

Vitex Agnus-castus

Vitex agnus-castus is a small shrub with yellow flowers and purple-red berries that grows in the Mediterranean region. It has been used for centuries as a traditional medicine for PMS, menstrual pain and irregularities, infertility, hormone imbalance, and menopause symptoms.

Vitex agnus-castus is a great essential oil for menopause. It can help with mood swings, hot flashes, and other symptoms. It also positively affects the body's endocrine system and can help balance out hormones. The scent of this essential oil is woody, earthy, and slightly citrus. It is often used in aromatherapy to help reduce stress levels, improve moods and increase energy levels.

- How it works

It is also known as Chaste Tree or Monk's Pepper because of its ability to calm sexual desire. Vitex agnus castus has an alkaloid called chastein that prevents ovulation by blocking the release of FSH (follicle-stimulating hormone). This helps balance estrogen levels in the body, reducing hot flashes and night sweats associated with menopause. In addition to reducing menopause symptoms, vitex agnus-castus also helps treat anxiety and depression, which are common during this time of life.

Sandalwood

Sandalwood is a very popular essential oil for menopause. It's known for its calming and cooling properties, which can help reduce hot flashes and night sweats. It's also been found to reduce anxiety, which can be common during menopause. Sandalwood essential oil is also antibacterial, so it can be used to keep the skin in good condition while you are going through the changes that come with menopause.

Ylang -ylang

Ylang-ylang is another great essential oil for menopause because it balances hormones and helps regulate the menstrual cycle by reducing symptoms like weight gain, mood swings, and cramps. This beautifully scented oil also has a calming effect on both mind and body which can help relieve some of those symptoms associated with menopause, such as hot flashes or night sweats, as well as anxiety caused by hormonal changes such as mood swings or depression from feeling left out. Ylang-ylang is an anti-inflammatory agent that helps reduce stress levels in your body and boost your immune system naturally so you can fight off any colds or infections that may come along during this time in your life.

Myrtle essential oil

Myrtle essential oil has been used for centuries to treat various menstrual disorders, including cramps and hot flashes. Myrtle can be used in diffuser blends or by applying it directly to the skin with a carrier oil. Myrtle essential oil is also known for promoting relaxation, so it's perfect for menopause-induced anxiety. It can be added to a bath or diffuser blend to reduce stress and

127

tension in the body.

The benefits of myrtle include:

-   Balancing estrogen levels in women with
    PMS or menopause
-   Helping regulate menstrual cycles and
    reduce hot flashes caused by hormone
    changes during menstrual cycles
-   Reducing anxiety and stress while
    promoting feelings of calmness and
    relaxation
-   Improving moods due to its uplifting
    properties using aromatherapy techniques
    such as massaging gently into the skin or
    inhaling from a diffuser near where you sit
    for an hour at least once daily during
    menopause symptoms

Yoga and Meditation

Yoga offers many benefits, including improved
flexibility and strength as well as increased vitality and
vigor (which will certainly be helpful during
menopause). Meditation has been shown to reduce
128

stress levels by releasing endorphins into the brain—these are chemicals that block pain signals from reaching other parts of the body, so it feels less tired after doing something stressful like working out at the gym!

Find Support

The experience of going through menopause can feel very isolating and may make you want to withdraw from friends and family and try and deal with things on your own. Although this is a normal reaction, after a while, it can often lead to feeling like everything is getting on top of you, and you might struggle to cope.

Find a family member or friend who is a good listener, doesn't judge you, makes you feel safe, and gives you the time and space to talk about your feelings. If you don't have someone like this, counseling can be beneficial. You can ask for this via your GP or find a counselor online.

As well as thinking about one-to-one counseling, being part of a network with people who have been through something similar can help reduce isolation and fear

129

and provide a supportive space. There are many relevant online chat forums and support groups.

CHAPTER 6: MENOPAUSE AT WORK

Many menopausal women find work stressful. You may find your productivity drops, and you're more easily distracted. You might also be less patient with co-workers who haven't had to deal with things like night sweats, night terrors, and hot flashes—which is why it's important to remember that menopause isn't just about hot flashes.

Women in the workplace have always faced a patchwork of policies and procedures that don't quite fit their needs. Take, for example, women who are in the middle of menopause. Its symptoms can make it difficult to focus on work and can even result in missed days at work.

Unfortunately, most workplaces don't yet have policies addressing this issue. While some employers offer paid sick leave or other accommodations for other medical conditions, they may not know how to handle a woman taking time off due to menopause symptoms. This can make it harder for employers who need to keep up with deadlines or simply want to keep their teams happy by keeping them healthy.

How to Manage Menopause at Work

Managing your menopause at work can be tricky, but there are several ways to make yourself more comfortable.

1) Talk about it with your boss.
2) Make sure you have enough time off when you need it.
3) Bring healthy snacks and drinks to look after your nutritional needs. Flasks of soup, jarred salads, or smoothies are good options. Avoid junk food or sweetened coffees from the

vending machines by always having a supply of your own snacks, such as nuts, dried fruit, and wholegrain crackers.

4) Schedule meetings early in the morning or at least before lunch so that if you feel tired later in the day it won't impact your ability to perform well at work.

5) Make sure you sleep well each night by going to bed earlier and getting up later. Practice good sleep hygiene principles, especially during the week.

6) Avoid caffeine after lunchtime and stop drinking alcohol three days before your period starts.

7) Keep your workspace cool by opening the windows or setting up fans on your desk. This will help reduce the symptoms of hot flashes and sweating. Keep a flask of iced water on your desk.

8) Dress in layers of comfortable, breathable fabrics. If you notice that wearing certain fabrics can make you feel hot or bothered, stick to cotton when possible. It's breathable and easy to wash. Dress in layers so that if you feel

too hot, you can strip off a few garments until you feel comfortable again.

9) Pay particular attention to your hygiene. When dealing with menopause symptoms like increased sweating, it's important to stay extra clean! Showering after work and again in the morning will help keep you smelling fresh and feeling confident about yourself at work. You may need to change to a stronger antiperspirant.

Is Menopause Derailing Your Career?

Menopause is a time of significant changes in a woman's life—and some of these can affect the way we work. Women can also find themselves struggling with memory loss, difficulty concentrating and multitasking, and other cognitive issues that can affect their ability to do their jobs well. If you're noticing any of these symptoms while at work, it might be time to talk to your doctor about how they could affect your ability to perform at peak capacity.

If you want to keep climbing the ladder, you need to

know how to handle menopause at work. Here are some tips for making it through this tricky stage:

1. Tell your boss about your symptoms
2. Take time off if you need it
3. Learn how to manage stress at work
4. Use reminder and organization tools such as apps, sticky notes, and alarms on your phone for deadlines

How to Speak to Your Manager and Co-workers about Menopause

Menopause is just a part of life; it doesn't have to be a big deal. Some people choose to keep it private, while others find it easier to discuss it with their manager and colleagues. Here are some tips for how to do that.

Start with yourself!

Begin by putting processes in place to help yourself at work, such as putting fans on your desk, providing healthy nutrition, and managing your deadlines well. Once you have done everything you can for yourself, it will give you more leverage when asking your boss and colleagues for concessions, such as a cooler air conditioner setting or time off work.

Be honest and open about your experience

Explain that you are going through a hormonal change right now and tell them that it may affect you emotionally and in other ways. Ask for patience but reassure everyone that you will still pull your weight in the team. Avoid using complicated medical jargon or going into detail about your ovaries!

Ask for help if you need it

If something isn't working out for you, don't be afraid to ask for advice from someone who knows more than you. Don't feel guilty about taking time off for yourself or medical appointments. It's not selfish—it's necessary!

Why Should Companies Be Taking Action to Support Menopause at Work?

Menopause can be tough on women who experience symptoms like hot flashes, night sweats, memory loss, and sleep disturbances. However, menopause doesn't just affect women—it affects the entire workplace. The more we understand the challenges that come with this transition, the better we can support one another and our colleagues.

We've listed some of the most common work challenges below:

-   Women in their 40s are usually hitting the peak of their careers, so having to deal with perimenopause and menopause can throw them off balance.
-   A survey by Fertifa and The Latte Lounge revealed that the most common symptoms relate to cognitive function, with 'brain fog' affecting nine out of 10 women going through menopause or perimenopause. Other common complaints were anxiety (84%) and depression (77%).
-   Studies have shown that perimenopause and menopause can have a significant impact on attendance and performance in the workplace. Untreated symptoms can be

wrongly identified as a performance issue. This is why communication about your condition is vital.

- Women are often at a higher risk for heart disease than men during menopause, so companies should take proactive measures to keep employees safe and perhaps provide access to screening measures.

- Women may need more time off because of their symptoms during the transition (like hormonal changes), which can take a toll on productivity if they don't feel empowered to talk about their needs openly with supervisors.

- Some women experience difficulty concentrating while going through menopause—which can affect their ability to perform well at work!

- There are many ways companies can support women during menopause:
  o Offer flexible hours and telecommuting options
  o Encourage employees to take breaks throughout the day

- ○ Provide bottled water and healthy snacks
- ○ Allow employees to wear comfortable clothing

Menopause can significantly affect your ability to perform at work. If you're experiencing menopause symptoms, it's not easy to think clearly or focus on work. That's why it's so important that businesses take action to support women who are going through menopause at work.

A Short Message from the Author

Hi, are you enjoying the book thus far? I'd love to hear your thoughts! Many readers do not know how hard reviews are to come by, and how much they help an author.

I would be incredibly thankful if you could take just 60 seconds to write a brief review, even if it's just a few sentences!

Thank you for taking the time to share your thoughts!

CHAPTER 7: BREAKING THE BIAS

As you might imagine, menopause can be quite stressful for women undergoing it—and not just because of the physical symptoms! Many women struggle with the idea that their bodies are no longer the same as they were before.

However, there's something else about menopause that isn't discussed enough: many people don't know what it is or how it works! This makes it hard for women to feel comfortable talking about their experiences and getting the support they need. So let's break down some common myths about menopause so we can all better understand what's happening in our bodies during this time and be able to explain it clearly to others.

Menopause is a topic often shrouded in mystery, stigma, and secrecy. Women are often afraid to talk about it for fear of being judged or because they think it's a "woman thing." But menopause isn't a woman's thing—it's a natural part of life that everyone needs to prepare for. Once when you're prepared, it can be an exciting time in your life! You can get more out of your body and mind and take advantage of new opportunities for personal growth.

Here are some things to know about menopause:

-       It's normal. Lots of people go through it! All women (apart from those who've had their ovaries removed before puberty) will experience menopause during their lifetime.
-       You don't have to go through it alone! There are many resources online and in person if you want help preparing yourself

mentally and physically for this time in your life.

- It can be very exhilarating. Think about all the cool things that happen when we're older than 40 and don't have to worry about having babies anymore—maybe we can start writing our memoirs!
- Menopause is a time of transition, but it's also a time of opportunity. You can take advantage of it to break free from the constraints of your old self and make way for the new person you're becoming.

Many negative stereotypes about menopause make women feel ashamed and embarrassed; they're afraid to talk about their experiences and what people will think of them if they do. There's a lot of talk in the workplace about the importance of flexibility, but sometimes it can feel like it doesn't apply to you. Maybe you've been told you must be available 24/7 and never get sick. Or maybe your boss has made comments about how "unprofessional" it is for you to take time off for doctor's appointments or family emergencies. It's time we changed this!

These things are frustrating—but they're also unfair.

Many women face barriers at work when they enter menopause due to outdated ideas about being a woman in her 50s and beyond. For example, if a woman is in her 50s and needs time off for treatment for a health issue related to menopause, she may be viewed as less capable than someone younger; or perhaps she will have trouble getting time off for annual check-ups because her boss doesn't understand that these are necessary during this time of life.

It's important to remember that women deserve respect and understanding no matter their age, even if their bodies have changed as part of their natural life experience! Did you know that one in four women consider dropping out of the workforce because of menopausal symptoms? This is shocking when you consider that most of those symptoms can be managed with a little extra effort and understanding.

Menopause doesn't mean you can't do your job

anymore. It doesn't mean you're no longer effective at work or that you're suddenly going to make mistakes all the time. It means that sometimes you might feel a little off-kilter because of hormonal changes—and that's okay! The truth is, menopause doesn't have to slow you down—it can help you become more productive!

Menopausal women are stereotyped as "experienced" but also "high risk and inefficient." This is the prevalent attitude of society towards these women, resulting in their exclusion from the workforce. However, this is not the case with menopause. Menopause is a natural process that affects everyone in one way or another, regardless of age, gender, and social status, because we are all linked.

Menopause affects every woman differently, but it does not mean they cannot lead a normal life or do their work efficiently during this phase. It is only for a short period that they need some extra support from their family members or colleagues at the workplace to get proper rest during this time.

We need to change our perception of menopause because it can be very stressful for women going through this phase in life. They may feel alienated from society because people don't understand what they are going through and make fun of them behind their backs!

There is an impact of the menopausal transition on women's relationships. For many women, the symptoms of menopause can be embarrassing and difficult to talk about. Women are often taught that it is not ladylike to show their emotions or to complain about their bodies. The shame, stigma, and lack of understanding that characterizes the menopausal transition can also impact intimate and intergenerational relationships.

It's Time to Break the Bias about Menopause

Menopause is a natural part of life in the same way that adolescence is, and yet we're surrounded by myths about it. From the idea that it's a taboo topic to the idea that it'll make you crazy, there are plenty of misconceptions out there. While some women may be able to ignore them, others feel as if their lives are falling apart as they struggle with symptoms like hot flashes, night sweats, and emotional rollercoasters.

However, there is a change afoot. A new, louder conversation about menopause is starting to take place. More women are educating themselves and their employers, speaking out instead of suffering in silence.

One example is the #MakeMenopauseMatter campaign, which is gaining support in the UK for menopause training for all GPs and workplace menopause policies. The campaign aims to raise awareness of how menopause affects women's lives at work and home by highlighting how it affects their productivity and mental health. It also asks employers to help their female employees by giving them information about what they can do to reduce its effects on them.

Silence on the topic can have a huge effect on women's lives, especially when they're at work. That's because some women suffer in silence. After all, they're afraid of losing their job or being treated differently if they raise the issue of their menopause with their employer. It doesn't have to be this way! There are things we can all do to break down these barriers and make sure that every woman has an equal chance at success during her menopausal years.

We need to talk about menopause

We must talk about it, educate ourselves, and raise awareness with friends and colleagues. We need to shift the shame and stigma around menopause and break this long-held taboo that discriminates against mid-aged women, enabling and empowering this undervalued group to thrive in our workplaces and contribute to our society fully.

CHAPTER 8: MOVING FORWARD IN THE POSTMENOPAUSE YEARS

Is there life after menopause?

Yes, Yes, and Yes!

After menopause, many women feel like they've lost their identity, but it doesn't have to be that way. You must understand why managing this transition is essential for your future health. Although this transition may seem overwhelming, there is a lot you can do to support your body, minimize the physical, mental, and emotional symptoms, and improve your overall health.

149

You are medically considered to be through menopause when you have not had a period for one year. By this time, your hormones should have found a new balance, and your body will likely have learned to cope with this new low level.

Many women feel just as good, if not better, after their periods have stopped – no more monthly blues, feeling low, bloating, etc., and as long as they continue to care for themselves, problems should not arise. Unfortunately, some women find that their menopause symptoms are not shifting even after this time and are wondering why.

The Power of Self-Acceptance

Know your menopause and own your menopause!

We all experience changes in our bodies during this time of life, which can be very different for each woman. However, it's important to remember that these changes are normal, just like other changes that occur throughout our lives, such as puberty, pregnancy, and childbirth.

150

When you're going through menopause, it's easy to feel like you've lost control. But what if we told you there is a way to take back some control?

We believe self-acceptance can help you take the reins and own your menopause.

Menopause is a natural process, so why do some women feel ashamed about it? The truth is that society has taught us to be ashamed of our bodies, especially when they are changing or when we go through changes like menopause. What if we could redefine what "normal" looks like? What if instead of seeing yourself as broken or flawed because of your changing body, you could see yourself as strong and capable? That's where self-acceptance comes in! Self-acceptance allows us to stop judging ourselves for who we are and what our bodies have been through. When we accept ourselves completely—all of our flaws and quirks—we can find true peace with who we are. And then we can start owning our menopause rather than letting it own us!

When we accept ourselves, we can stop trying to be

someone else. This means no more trying to be younger than we are—no more spending hours in front of the mirror and worrying about our wrinkles or gray hair! When we accept ourselves, it's easier for us to let go of those external factors that make us feel insecure or unhappy about ourselves.

The Power of Self-Care

It's easy to get caught up in the negativity of menopause and feel like you're just not good enough anymore. However, it's important to remember that you are more than your age, and every woman goes through this at some point in their life.

Take a moment to think about what makes you a strong person—what makes you who you are? Is it your family? Your friends? Your career? What are the things that bring meaning into your life? Think about these things, and write them down. Then, create new rules and beliefs that help support those positive traits. For example: "I am strong because I have a supportive family" or "I am kind because I surround myself with kind people."

When you start feeling down about yourself or menopause, remind yourself of these new rules and beliefs so that it becomes second nature!

Here are some tips for creating new rules and beliefs about menopause:

1) Make peace with your body. Accept that it has changed since you were young and that those changes are normal and you can still be beautiful.

2) Be kind to yourself. Give yourself credit for what you do well, even if it's not perfect!

3) Remember that this is just one stage of your life— and many other phases are waiting for you!

Manage Self-destructive thoughts

If you're having self-destructive thoughts about menopause, you're not alone. Menopause can be a confusing and even scary time. Your body is changing, and it's not just about your periods. You might find that you suddenly have hot flashes or your skin's quality has changed. These changes can make us feel

153

like we're losing control over our bodies and lives!

Focus on what works for you

Menopause isn't a one-size-fits-all experience; everyone handles it differently! So if you have found something that works for you and makes it easier to get through this time, then keep doing it! If something isn't working for you, try something else until you find something that works well enough to help with those feelings of losing control over your body/life.

Self-Care

One of the most important steps you can take during menopause is to make time for yourself. It is also probably one of the hardest! As women, menopause should be a time when we rest and allow our bodies to adapt to all the hormonal changes.

Treat yourself to something nice—a massage or pedicure, perhaps—and take some time out for yourself every day or two so you don't become overwhelmed by all the changes in your body and mind.

It also helps to remember that we're not alone in this journey! Other women have gone through it too, and many of them have found ways to cope with their experiences. So don't feel alone—others have felt what you're feeling now and have managed it successfully!

Meditation

Meditation is excellent for women who want to reduce their stress, anxiety, and depression during this transition. Meditation helps to reduce the intensity of negative emotions and teaches you to focus on your breathing. It can help you relax, feel less stressed, and be more focused daily.

Meditation helps with this by increasing awareness of your body's signals about how you're feeling—your heart rate or breathing patterns may change depending on what's happening around you or how much stress is mounting up inside your body. Awareness of these signs can give clues as to whether or not something is going wrong with how well your body is handling its transition into menopause.

Affirmations

Menopause is a topic that people often feel sensitive about. Affirmations are a great way to overcome this discomfort by acknowledging the positive side of it.

For example, proclaim:

"I am strong."

"I am confident."

"I am beautiful."

"I have a strong body."

"I am resilient and can adapt to change."

"I will not be defined by my hormones but by my strength and self-control."

"I am thankful for life."

"I am grateful."

The Power of Gratitude

Gratitude is a powerful force for good. It can change your life and make you happier, healthier, and more connected to the people around you. But what if there was a way to use gratitude as a tool for change during menopause?

That's right—gratitude can be used during menopause to help reduce symptoms like hot flashes, mood swings, and night sweats. The best part is that it doesn't require any additional time or effort on your part; all you have to do is be grateful!

The key is in knowing exactly what you're grateful for. For example, if you're having trouble sleeping at night because of hot flashes, be grateful for the fact that your partner can stay up with you until they pass or go back down to normal levels again. You could also be thankful that he doesn't mind being woken up every few hours by your condition (and will even make sure he gets up with you so that both of you get some sleep!). If this sounds like something you could use in your marriage relationship right now—start thanking him every time he wakes up so he knows just how much it means to you.

How can you use this to your advantage? By being grateful for all the things that make life worth living! Take time each day to think about what makes you happy and remember those things when times get tough. You'll be surprised by how much better you feel when you're able to look back on all the good things in your life with appreciation instead of taking them for granted!

CONCLUSION

Menopause is a natural process that happens to every woman, and it's nothing to be afraid of. However, it's time to talk to your doctor if you're struggling with symptoms like hot flashes, night sweats, mood swings, or trouble sleeping.

If you're suffering from these symptoms, ensure you're eating right and getting enough exercise. If that doesn't help, talk to your doctor about how medication could help make menopause easier on you. Menopause is an exciting time in your life. It's the end of one chapter and the beginning of another!

My aim for this book was to demystify menopause and explain in simple terms what may happen to you and how you can help yourself through this stage of life as easily as possible. I want you to remember that the key to an easier menopause transition is maintaining good overall health – and this doesn't have to be complicated!

You've come a long way and are ready to take on new challenges. You should feel proud of how far you've come, but don't let that stop you from setting new goals for yourself. You've already reached a milestone by making it through menopause—now set some new goals. Take up a new hobby, learn something new about yourself, or volunteer for a cause that inspires you. You'll be surprised by how much more confident you feel when you're doing things that make you happy!

One more thing

If you enjoyed this book and found it helpful, I'd be very grateful if you'd post a short review on Amazon. Your support does make a difference, and I read all the reviews personally so I can get your feedback and make this book even better. I love hearing from my readers, and I'd really appreciate it if you leave your honest feedback.

Thank you for reading!

Bonus Chapter

I would like to share a sneak peek into another one of my books that I think you will enjoy. The book is titled ***"Women with ADHD Falling through the Cracks: Unmasking the Bias and Exploring Why ADD and ADHD Symptoms in Adult Women and Girls Are Misunderstood and Undiagnosed."***

Women with attention-deficit/hyperactivity disorder (ADHD) are falling through the cracks, and it's time to talk about it.

ADHD is not just a problem for kids and

163

males. With centuries of cultural stereotypes about women's supposed lack of intellect, women with ADHD are often overlooked and unacknowledged. **50%-75% of ADHD cases in females are missed.** This diagnosis gap happens partly because it's a condition that was traditionally thought to affect mostly men, but also because women tend to have less obvious or socially disruptive symptoms than men. Males tend to be diagnosed more often and sooner because their symptoms are usually more physical and obvious. Inattentive ADHD, the most common ADHD presentation in females, tends to be mental rather than physical. Since many of these symptoms take place inside the mind, they can be easy for parents, patients and mental health professionals to miss.

ADHD is a challenging condition for women and girls. According to the Centers for Disease Control and Prevention, the diagnosis rate among females is 40% lower than males. The symptoms can be different but the consequences are just as serious. Women with ADHD often go undiagnosed or misdiagnosed, which negatively impacts their mental & physical wellbeing and relationships. The good news? ADHD can be managed with medication and coaching. This book introduces ADHD through the lens of women, offers tips for managing daily life, and includes a list of resources for women in particular.

This book will teach you:

- What is ADHD

- How to diagnose ADHD

- ADHD management strategies

- Tips for parents of an ADHD child

- Treatment options of ADHD

- How ADHD symptoms differs in women

- Why ADHD Is Underdiagnosed in Women

- Challenges of women with ADHD

If you are a woman with ADHD, you should know that it is a very treatable condition. As overwhelmed as you may feel, know that you can feel better. There is a lot you can do to regain control of your life, instead of having ADHD control you.

It's time to Know Your ADHD and Own Your ADHD!

Enjoy this free chapter!

The majority of research on attention deficit hyperactivity disorder (ADHD) has traditionally focused on males, who were believed to make up 80% of all those with ADHD. Now more and more females are being identified, especially now that we are more aware of the non-hyperactive subtype of ADHD. Girls and women with ADHD struggle with a variety of issues that are different from those faced by males. This book will highlight some of those differences, and we will explore the types of struggles faced by females with ADHD.

ADHD is a neurodevelopmental disorder characterized by impulsive behavior and related symptoms. The disorder is classified into three types: impulsive/hyperactivity, inattention/distractibility, and a combination.

While ADHD is the most common disorder among

boys aged four to eleven, only about half as many girls are diagnosed, according to the Australian Institute of Health and Welfare. While women tend to develop ADHD later in life, most symptoms appear in infancy and go undiagnosed, untreated, or are well-masked by social and communication abilities.

According to Mark Bellgrove, a professor of cognitive neuroscience, females with ADHD are more likely than males to abuse substances. He stated, "As a result, we want to catch them sooner and treat them more effectively. However, I believe it is safe to say they are slipping through the cracks."

According to some studies, up to three-quarters of adult women with ADHD are undiagnosed. Many women diagnosed with ADHD as adults reflect on the red flags they ignored as children, such as difficulties in school or difficulties making friends. They wonder how their lives would have changed if their condition had been identified earlier. Coping with symptoms becomes more difficult for those not diagnosed as their responsibilities grow in adulthood.

According to ADHD-specialist psychologist Tamara May, some women receive an ADHD diagnosis after years of struggling with symptoms of "secondary" depression and anxiety due to the problem not being diagnosed. "During adolescence, many women realize they are struggling more than their classmates, but they don't know why," she adds. People underestimate the severity of ADHD and how difficult even the most basic tasks can be. "You're being lazy; you should be able to do better," people around them say. Simply getting up and doing the dishes can be a challenge.

This medical issue is exacerbated by the fact that there are a limited number of psychiatrists who specialize in

169

ADHD, almost all of whom work in the private sector. According to Dr. May, it is extremely rare for someone to be diagnosed in the public hospital system. "Women must first recognize that they are experiencing symptoms of ADHD before consulting with their primary care physician and obtaining a referral to see a private psychiatrist. Waitlists range from three to six months, and some psychiatrists have closed their doors." Some women have reported spending up to $2,000 to get a diagnosis confirmed.

Furthermore, obtaining ADHD medication necessitates a consultation with a psychiatrist. Women who want to change their lives by recognizing and accepting their ADHD must take the initiative. While public awareness of adult ADHD is growing, research biases persist. Women's specific complications such as the effects of pregnancy, menopause, hormones, and the menstrual cycle on ADHD symptoms have received little attention.

Women are just as negatively affected by ADHD as men, if not more so. While most ADHD research has focused on white male participants, some studies have included or focused on the life outcomes of adult female ADHD patients. This book does a detailed analysis and provides helpful solutions.

ADHD is a disorder with a high comorbidity rate. It has been determined that ADHD in a girl or woman increases the likelihood that she will experience trauma at some point in her life. The most common comorbid diagnoses in women are depression, anxiety, and eating disorders. While these diagnoses frequently co-occur, it has been discovered that many women are misdiagnosed with conditions such as anxiety or depression when the underlying issue is ADHD. Unintended pregnancies, marital abuse, and an

171

increased risk of self-harm and suicide are more common in women with ADHD than in the general population. While the literature indicates that living with ADHD hurts both men and women, gender differences among people with ADHD have not been thoroughly investigated. However, this research is necessary because the number of women diagnosed with ADHD has risen in recent years. This is partly due to practitioners' increased awareness that not only can ADHD persist into adulthood, but it is also not a gender-based illness.

Women whose disabilities or struggles may have gone unnoticed or been misinterpreted during childhood and adolescence struggle to cope with the inevitable increase in adult responsibilities. This trend has been picked up and written about in the popular press. Many doctors and psychiatrists agree that a lack of research is a problem. They believe that advances in this area could reduce stigma and provide greater inclusion for people with ADHD and other illnesses.

Despite the bad press and lack of research, there are success stories. Ms. Josie Bober's is one. Despite consistently high grades, Ms. Bober had been unable to complete any of the university degrees she had begun before her diagnosis. Despite her illness, she recently completed a graphic design degree and is now determined to help others by making universities more welcoming to neurodiverse people. Her alma mater, the University of New South Wales, has even provided her with funding to conduct workshops with students and professors to develop effective strategies. In her interview, she stated, "I was feeling proactive. I believe I reached a point within myself where I felt confident and eager to help others. "Increased ADHD diagnoses among women should improve their overall performance and quality of life. However, a lack of

173

research on women with ADHD may result in gender-specific requirements and overlooked obstacles in this population."

This book offers a comprehensive insight into the identification, treatment, and support for girls and women with ADHD. It is critical to reject the widely held belief that ADHD is a behavioral disorder and concentrate on the more subtle and internalized presentation typical of females. Adopting a lifelong model of care is critical to assist the multiple transitions that females experience concurrently with changes in their clinical presentation and social situations. Treatment with pharmacological and psychological therapies is expected to increase productivity, reduce resource use, and, most importantly, better the long-term outcomes for girls and women. This book is a must-have for any girl or woman who thinks she may have ADHD!